Acne Scars

Series in Dermatological Treatment
Published in association with the *Journal of Dermatological Treatment*
Series editors: *Steven R Feldman and Peter van de Kerkhof*

Acne Scars

Classification and Treatment

Edited by

Antonella Tosti, MD
Department of Dermatology
University of Bologna
Bologna
Italy

Maria Pia De Padova, MD
Department of Dermatology
Nigrisoli Private Hospital
Bologna
Italy

Kenneth R Beer, MD
Palm Beach Esthetic Center
West Palm Beach, Florida
USA

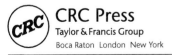

CRC Press
Taylor & Francis Group
Boca Raton   London   New York

CRC Press is an imprint of the
Taylor & Francis Group, an **informa** business

CRC Press
Taylor & Francis Group
6000 Broken Sound Parkway NW, Suite 300
Boca Raton, FL 33487-2742

First issued in paperback 2019

© 2010 by Taylor & Francis Group, LLC
CRC Press is an imprint of Taylor & Francis Group, an Informa business

No claim to original U.S. Government works

ISBN-13: 978-1-84184-687-3 (hbk)
ISBN-13: 978-0-367-38471-5 (pbk)

This book contains information obtained from authentic and highly regarded sources. While all reasonable efforts have been made to publish reliable data and information, neither the author[s] nor the publisher can accept any legal responsibility or liability for any errors or omissions that may be made. The publishers wish to make clear that any views or opinions expressed in this book by individual editors, authors or contributors are personal to them and do not necessarily reflect the views/opinions of the publishers. The information or guidance contained in this book is intended for use by medical, scientific or health-care professionals and is provided strictly as a supplement to the medical or other professional's own judgement, their knowledge of the patient's medical history, relevant manufacturer's instructions and the appropriate best practice guidelines. Because of the rapid advances in medical science, any information or advice on dosages, procedures or diagnoses should be independently verified. The reader is strongly urged to consult the relevant national drug formulary and the drug companies' and device or material manufacturers' printed instructions, and their websites, before administering or utilizing any of the drugs, devices or materials mentioned in this book. This book does not indicate whether a particular treatment is appropriate or suitable for a particular individual. Ultimately it is the sole responsibility of the medical professional to make his or her own professional judgements, so as to advise and treat patients appropriately. The authors and publishers have also attempted to trace the copyright holders of all material reproduced in this publication and apologize to copyright holders if permission to publish in this form has not been obtained. If any copyright material has not been acknowledged please write and let us know so we may rectify in any future reprint.

A CIP record for this book is available from the British Library.

Library of Congress Cataloging-in-Publication Data available on application

Visit the Taylor & Francis Web site at
http://www.taylorandfrancis.com

and the CRC Press Web site at
http://www.crcpress.com

Contents

v

List of contributors

Murad Alam
Department of Dermatology
Northwestern University
Chicago, Illinois, USA

Saba M Ali
Department of Dermatology
Wake Forest University School of Medicine
Winston-Salem, North Carolina, USA

Mauro Barbareschi
Institute of Dermatological Sciences, University of
    Milan
IRCCS Foundation
and Ospedale Maggiore Policlinico, Mangiagalli and
    Regina Elena
Milan, Italy

Kenneth R Beer
Palm Beach Esthetic Center
West Palm Beach, Florida, USA

James Q Del Rosso
Mohave Skin & Cancer Clinics
Las Vegas, Nevada USA
Valley Hospital Medical Center
Las Vegas, Nevada USA

Maria Pia De Padova
Department of Dermatology
Nigrisoli Private Hospital
Bologna, Italy

Gabriella Fabbrocini
Department of Dermatology
University of Naples
Naples, Italy

Nunzio Fardella
Department of Dermatology
University of Naples
Naples, Italy

Timothy Corcoran Flynn
Cary Skin Center
Cary, North Carolina
and Department of Dermatology
University of North Carolina
Chapel Hill, North Carolina, USA

Lidia Francesconi
Dermatology Clinic
University of Catania
Catania, Italy

Ma Teresita G Gabriel
Research Institute for Tropical Medicine
Department of Health
Metro Manila, Philippines

Evangeline B Handog
Research Institute for Tropical Medicine
Department of Health
and Department of Dermatology
Asian Hospital and Medical Center
Metro Manila, Philippines

Christopher B Harmon
Surgical Dermatology Group
Birmingham, Alabama, USA

†Daniele Innocenzi
Department of Dermatology
University of Rome I
Rome, Italy

Ravneet R Kaur
Department of Dermatology
Wake Forest University School of Medicine
Winston-Salem, North Carolina, USA

Grace K Kim
Mohave Skin & Cancer Clinics
Las Vegas, Nevada USA

Francesco Lacarrubba
Dermatology Clinic
University of Catania
Catania, Italy

Marina Landau
Department of Dermatology
Wolfson Medical Center
Holon, Israel

Ma Juliet E Macarayo
Angeles University Foundation Medical Center
Angeles City, Pampanga, Philippines

Amy J McMichael
Department of Dermatology
Wake Forest University School of Medicine
Winston-Salem, North Carolina, USA

Giuseppe Micali
Dermatology Clinic
University of Catania
Catania, Italy

Maria Miteva
Department of Dermatology and Cutaneous Suurgery
University of Miami Miller School of Medicine
Miami, Florida, USA

Ambra Monfrecola
Department of Dermatology
University of Naples
Naples, Italy

Beatrice Nardone
Dermatology Clinic
University of Catania
Catania, Italy

Vic A Narurkar
Bay Area Laser Institute
and California Pacific Medical Center
San Francisco, California
and Department of Dermatology
University of California at Davis School of Medicine
Davis, California, USA

Megan Pirigyi
Department of Dermatology
Northwestern University
Chicago, Illinois, USA

Ilaria Proietti
Department of Dermatology
University of Rome I
Rome, Italy

Paolo Romanelli
Department of Dermatology and Cutaneous Surgery
University of Miami Miller School of Medicine
Miami, Florida, USA

Aurora Tedeschi
Department of Dermatology
University of Catania
Catania
Italy

Jens J Thiele
Dermatology Specialists, Inc.
Oceanside, California, USA

Antonella Tosti
Department of Dermatology
University of Bologna
Bologna, Italy

Stefano Veraldi
Institute of Dermatological Sciences
University of Milan
and IRCCS Foundation
Ospedale Maggiore Policlinico,
    Mangiagalli and Regina Elena
Milan, Italy

Lee E West
Pharmacy Department
Northwestern Memorial Hospital
Chicago
and
Department of Dermatology
Northwestern University
Chicago, Illinois, USA

1 Classification of acne scars: A review with clinical and ultrasound correlation

Giuseppe Micali, Lidia Francesconi, Beatrice Nardone, and Francesco Lacarrubba

INTRODUCTION

Scar is defined as "the fibrous tissue that replaces normal tissue destroyed by injury or disease".(1) Causes of acne scar formation can be broadly categorized as either the result of increased tissue formation or, more commonly, loss or damage of local tissue.(2)

Clinical manifestations of acne scars as well as severity of scarring are generally related to the degree of inflammatory reaction, to tissue damage, and to time lapsed since the onset of tissue inflammation.(3, 4) There have been attempts to classify acne scars in order to standardize severity assessments and treatment modalities.(3, 4) However, consensus concerning acne scar nomenclature and classification is still lacking.(3)

CLINICAL CLASSIFICATIONS

In 1987 Ellis et al. proposed an acne scar classification system and utilized the descriptive terms ice pick, crater, undulation, tunnel, shallow-type, and hypertrophic scars.(5) Langdon, in 1999, distinguished three types of acne scars: Type 1, shallow scars that are small in diameter; Type 2, ice pick scars; and Type 3, distensible scars.(6) Lately, Goodman et al. proposed that atrophic acne scars may be divided into superficial macular, deeper dermal, perifollicular scarring, and fat atrophy based on pathophysiologic features.(7)

One classification system frequently used in clinical practice for acne scars is based on both clinical and histological features.(8) Acne scars are classified into three basic types depending on width, depth, and 3-dimensional architecture:

- *Icepick scars:* narrow (diameter < 2 mm), deep, sharply marginated and depressed tracks that extend vertically to the deep dermis or subcutaneous tissue.
- *Boxcar scars:* round to oval depressions with sharply demarcated vertical edges. They are wider at the surface than icepick scars and do not taper to a point at the base. These scars may be shallow (0.1–0.5 mm) or deep (≥ 0.5 mm) and the diameter may vary from 1.5 to 4.0 mm.
- *Rolling scars:* occur from dermal tethering of otherwise relatively normal-appearing skin and are usually wider than 4 to 5 mm in diameter. An abnormal fibrous anchoring of the dermis to the subcutis leads to superficial shadowing and to a rolling or undulating appearance of the overlying skin.

Other clinical entities included in this classification are *hypertrophic scars, keloidal scars,* and *sinus tracts.*(8) Both hypertrophic and keloidal scars result from an abnormal excessive tissue repair: clinically, hypertrophic scars are raised within the limits of primary excision, whereas keloidal scars transgress this boundary and may show prolonged and continuous growth. (9) Sinus tracts may appear as grouped open comedones histologically showing a number of interconnecting keratinized channels.(7)

Another classification is that proposed by Kadunc et al.(3) Based on clinical appearance and relationship to surrounding skin, acne scars are classified in this system as elevated, dystrophic, or depressed. Other parameters include shape, consistency, colour, and distensibility. This classification system may also serve to assess the efficacy of various therapeutic options based on acne scars types.(3) Kadunc's classification is summarized in Table 1.1.

Goodman et al. proposed a qualitative grading system that differentiates four grades according to scar severity (Table 1.2): Grade I corresponds to macular involvement (including erythematous, hyperpigmented, or hypopigmented scars), whereas Grades II, III, and IV correspond to mild, moderate, and severe atrophic and hypertrophic lesions, respectively. (10) Interestingly, the authors consider lesion severity also according to visibility at a social distance (≥ 50 cm). Moreover, since patients may present various types of acne scars at numerous anatomic sites (i.e., one cheek, the neck, the chest, and so on; these single areas are defined by the authors as "cosmetic units"), scars are further subdivided into four grades of severity by anatomic sites involved, and the localized disease (up to three involved areas) is classified as A (focal, 1 cosmetic unit involvement) or B (discrete, 2–3 cosmetic units), whereas the involvement of more cosmetic units is classified as generalized disease, previously described in Table 1.2.

The same authors subsequently, suggested a quantitative numeric grading system based on lesion counting (1–10, 11–20, >20), scar type (atrophic, macular, boxcar, hypertrophic, keloidal), and severity (mild, moderate, severe). Final scoring depends on the addition of points assigned to each respective category and reflects disease severity, ranging from a minimum of 0 to a maximum of 84 (Table 1.3).(11)

Finally, Dreno et al. first proposed the ECLA scale (echelle d'evaluation clinique des lesions d'acne) (12), followed by the ECCA grading scale (echelle d'evaluation clinique des cicatrices d'acne) (4). According to this scoring system, morphological aspects of lesions define the type of scars as

Table 1.1 Kadunc's morphologic classification of acne scars.

Scars Types	Clinical Description
1. Elevated	
1a. Hypertrophic	Hypertrophic lesions raised above the skin surface and limited to the original injured area
1b. Keloidal	Usually found in patients with genetic predisposition; their dimensions exceed the initial injured tissue
1c. Papular	Soft elevations, like anetodermas, frequently observed on the trunk and chin area
1d. Bridges	Fibrous strings over healthy skin
2. Dystrophic	Irregular or star-like scar shapes with a white and atrophic floor
3. Depressed	
3a.1. Distensible retractions	Scars attached only by their central area after skin distension
3a.2. Distensible undulations (valleys)	Lesion that do not completely disappear after skin distension
3b.1. Nondistensible superficial	Shallow, dish-like defects
3b.2. Nondistensible medium	Crater like, with a scar base that is relatively smooth and has normal color and texture and wide diameter
3b.3. Nondistensible deep	Narrow and fibrotic scars, ice-pick or pitted scars with sharp shoulders perpendicular to the skin surface that may appear as epithelial invaginations sometimes reaching the subcutaneous layer
3b.4. Tunnels	Two or more ice-pick scars connected by epithelialized tracts

Source: Kadunc BV et al. (3).

Table 1.2 Goodman's qualitative global scarring grading system.

Grade	Level of Disease	Clinical Features	Examples of Scars
1	Macular disease	Erythematous, hyper- or hypo-pigmented flat marks visible to patient or observer irrespective of distance	Erythematous, hyper- or hypo-pigmented flat marks
2	Mild disease	Mild atrophy or hypertrophy that may not be obvious at social distances of 50 cm or greater and may be covered adequately by makeup or the normal shadow of shaved beard hair in males or normal body hair if extrafacial	Mild rolling, small soft papular
3	Moderate disease	Moderate atrophic or hypertrophic scarring that is obvious at social distances of 50 cm or greater and is not covered easily by makeup or the normal shadow of shaved beard hair in males or body hair if extrafacial, but is still able to be flattened by manual stretching of the skin	More significant rolling, shallow "box car," mild to moderate hypertrophic or papular scars
4	Severe disease	Severe atrophic or hypertrophic scarring that is obvious at social distances of 50 cm or greater and is not covered easily by makeup or the normal shadow of shaved beard hair in males or body hair (if extrafacial) and is not able to be flattened by manual stretching of the skin	Punched out atrophic (deep "box car"), "ice pick", bridges and tunnels, gross atrophy, dystrophic scars, significant hypertrophy or keloid

Source: Goodman GJ et al. (10).

follows: atrophic scars (V-shaped, U-shaped and M-shaped), superficial elastolysis, hypertrophic inflammatory scars (<2 years since onset), and keloid-hypertrophic scars (>2 years since onset). Each scar type is associated with a quantitative score (0, 1, 2, 3 depending on the number of lesions) multiplied by a weighting factor that varies according to severity, evolution, and morphological aspect. The final global score is directly correlated with clinical severity and ranges from 0 to 540 depending on the type and number of acne scars (Table 1.4).

CLINICAL AND ULTRASOUND CORRELATIONS

Methods

Ultrasound imaging is a noninvasive technique that uses various acoustic properties of biologic tissues. Typically, echo signals are represented in one-dimensional diagrams (A-mode) or two-dimensional images (B-mode).

Ultrasound of the skin is best performed by equipment using frequencies of $\geq$ 20 MHz. Using B-mode imaging, normal skin typically shows an epidermal entrance echo, the

Table 1.3 Goodman's quantitative global acne scarring grading system.

Grade or Type	Number of Lesions 1 (1–10)	Number of Lesions 2 (11–20)	Number of Lesions 3 (>20)
A) **Milder scarring** (1 point each) Macular erythematous or pigmented Mildly atrophic dish-like	1 point	2 points	3 points
B) **Moderate scarring** (2 points each) Moderately atrophic, dish like Punched out with shallow bases small scars (<5 mm) Shallow but broad atrophic areas	2 points	4 points	6 points
C) **Severe scarring** (3 points each) Punched out with deep but normal bases, small scars (<5 mm) Punched out with deep abnormal bases, small scars (<5 mm) Linear or troughed dermal scarring Deep, broad atrophic areas	3 points	6 points	9 points
D) **Hyperplastic** Papular scars Keloidal/hypertrophic scars	2 points Area < 5 mm 6 points	4 points Area 5–20 cm^2 12 points	6 points Area > 20 cm^2 18 points

Source: Goodman GJ et al. (11).

Table 1.4 ECCA grading scale.

Description	Weighting Factor (a)	Semiquantitative Score (b)	Grading (a × b)
V-shaped atrophic scars, diameter of less than 2 mm, and punctiform	15	0 = no scar 1 = a few scars 2 = limited number of scars 3 = many scars	/_____/
U-shaped atrophic scars, diameter of 2–4 mm, with sheer edges	20	0 = no scar 1 = a few scars 2 = limited number of scars 3 = many scars	/_____/
M-shaped atrophic scars, diameter of more than 4 mm, superficial and with irregular surface	25	0 = no scar 1 = a few scars 2 = limited number of scars 3 = many scars	/_____/
Superficial elastolysis	30	0 = no scar 1 = a few scars 2 = limited number of scars 3 = many scars	/_____/
Subgrading 1			/_____/
Hypertrophic inflammatory scars, scars of less than 2 years of age	40	0 = no scar 1 = a few scars 2 = limited number of scars 3 = many scars	/_____/
Keloid scars and hypertrophic scars that are more than 2 years of age	50	0 = no scar 1 = a few scars 2 = limited number of scars 3 = many scars	/_____/
Subgrading 2			/_____/
Global Score (Subgrading 1 + 2)			/_____/

Source: Dreno B et al. (4).

dermal layer, and the subcutaneous layer. This technique offers a wide range of possibilities in clinical and experimental dermatology. It is used for the evaluation of skin tumour thickness (e.g., basal-cell carcinoma, melanoma). Areas of research may include scleroderma, psoriasis, and aged and photoaged skin. Moreover, it provides an objective measurement of skin thickness and has been utilized to assess thickness of hypertrophic scars before and after treatment.(13)

A preliminary study was preformed in a series of patients ($N = 20$) affected by various types of acne scars in order to determine whether a correlation exists between clinical appearance of selected scar parameters (thickness, width, depth) with ultrasound examination. Cross-sectional B-mode scans were obtained using a 22-MHz ultrasound system (EasyScan Echo®, Business Enterprise, Trapani, Italy) that allowed examination of skin sections of 12 mm in width and 8 mm in depth.

Results

- ***Atrophic scars*** appear as invaginations of the skin in which all skin layers are normally represented:

  a) *Icepick scars* ($n = 5$) uniformly have a sharp, demarcated V-shaped appearance and are characterized by a narrow diameter at the surface (usually < 2 mm) and

a vertical extension that reaches a depth corresponding to the deep dermis (Figure 1.1a–1.1b).

  b) *Boxcar scars* ($n = 5$) uniformly present with a sharp demarcated U-shaped appearance and are characterized by a superficial diameter usually ranging from 2 to 4 mm and a vertical extension that reaches a depth corresponding to the superficial or deep dermis (Figure 1.2a–1.2b).

  c) *Rolling scars* ($n = 5$) uniformly appear as large (up to 5 mm) poorly demarcated depressions of the skin; these scars are very superficial, sometimes hardly visible, with a vertical extension that is limited to a depth corresponding to the epidermal thickness (Figure 1.3a–1.3b).

- ***Hypertrophic and keloidal scars*** ($n = 5$) uniformly appear as dome-shaped, localized increase of skin thickness (Figure 4a–4b; 5a–5b); the dermis usually is less echogenic than normal skin; in most cases, with the 22 MHz probe, keloidal scars may not be entirely visualized because of their large size.

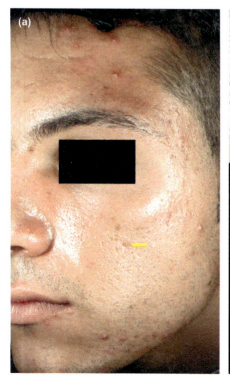

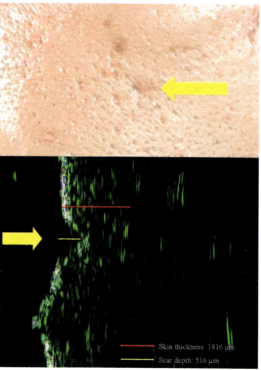

Skin thickness: 1816 μm
Scar depth: 516 μm

Figure 1.1 Icepick scar: clinical and ultrasound appearance.

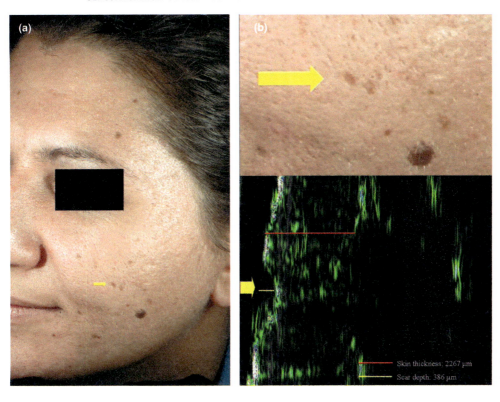

Figure 1.2 Boxcar scar: clinical and ultrasound appearance.

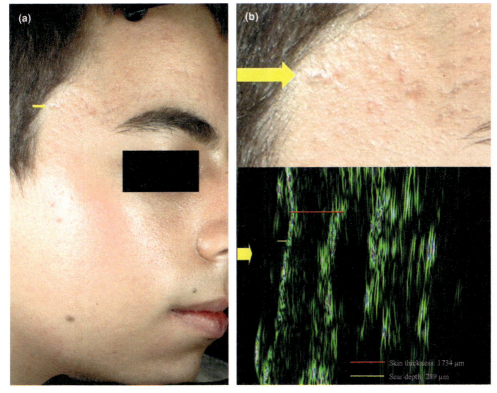

Figure 1.3 Rolling scar: clinical and ultrasound appearance.

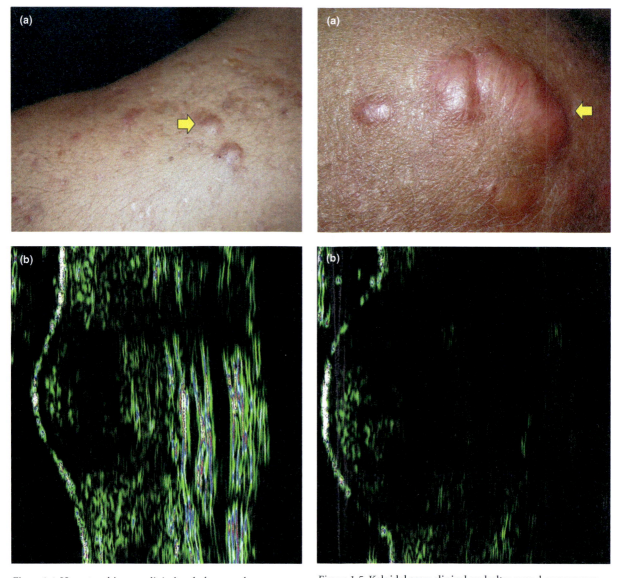

Figure 1.4 Hypertrophic scar: clinical and ultrasound appearance.

Figure 1.5 Keloidal scar: clinical and ultrasound appearance.

CONCLUSIONS

There is a lack of consensus in the literature regarding acne scar nomenclature and classification. A major problem is represented by the pleomorphic appearance of scars that may cause variable interpretation at clinical examination. A standard method for evaluation of scar depth represents an unmet need and is essential for therapeutic and prognostic purposes. Ultrasound examination provides simple and reproducible quantitative parameters, representing a promising tool for a more accurate evaluation and classification of acne scars.

REFERENCES

1. "Scar." The American Heritage® Stedman's Medical Dictionary. Houghton Mifflin Company. 10 Feb. 2009. Available from: http://dictionary.reference.com/browse/scar.
2. Rivera AE. Acne scarring: a review and current treatment modalities. J Am Acad Dermatol 2008; 59: 659–76.
3. Kadunc BV, Trindade de Almeida AD. Surgical treatment of facial acne scars based on morphologic classification: a Brazilian experience. Dermatol Surg 2003; 29: 1200–9.

4. Dreno B, Khammari A, Orain N et al. ECCA grading scale: an original validated acne scar grading scale for clinical practice in dermatology. Dermatology 2007; 214: 46–51.

5. Ellis DA, Michell MJ. Surgical treatment of acne scarring: non-linear scar revision. J Otolaryngol 1987; 16: 2116–9.

6. Langdon RC. Regarding dermabrasion for acne scars [letter]. Dermatol Surg 1999; 25: 919–20.

7. Goodman GJ. Postacne scarring: a review of its pathophysiology and treatment. Dermatol Surg 2000; 26: 857–71.

8. Jacob CI, Dover JS, Kaminer MS. Acne scarring: a classification system and review of treatment options. J Am Acad Dermatol 2001; 45: 109–17.

9. Jemec GB, Jemec B. Acne: treatment of scars. Clin Dermatol 2004; 22: 434–8.

10. Goodman GJ, Baron JA. Postacne scarring: a qualitative global scarring grading system. Dermatol Surg 2006; 32: 1458–66.

11. Goodman GJ, Baron JA. Postacne scarring–a quantitative global scarring grading system. J Cosmet Dermatol 2006; 5: 48–52.

12. Dreno B, Bodokh I, Chivot M et al. ECLA grading: a system of acne classification for every day dermatological practice. Ann Dermatol Venereol 1999; 126: 136–41.

13. Lacarrubba F, Patania L, Perrotta R et al. An open-label pilot study to evaluate the efficacy and tolerability of a silicone gel in the treatment of hypertrophic scars using clinical and ultrasound assessments. J Dermatol Treat 2008; 19: 50–3.

2 Pathophysiology of acne scars
Stefano Veraldi and Mauro Barbareschi

INTRODUCTION
Scars can affect a high percentage of patients with acne and can occur early. Two features in scar development are important: (a) its severity, and (b) the delay before an adequate treatment. It is, therefore, important to inform patients with inflammatory acne (from papular-pustular to nodular-cystic) that they have a high risk of scar development.(1)

Dermoepidermal wound is characterized by a cascade of events that culminate in scar development at the site of tissue damage. Morphology of scars varies among patients: This variability depends on intrinsic and extrinsic factors, resulting in the development of a normal or a pathologic scar.

Inspite of the knowledge gathered via research so far, exact mechanisms of damaged tissue healing remain poorly understood, particularly about pathological scars.

PHYSIOLOGICAL WOUND HEALING AND SCAR DEVELOPMENT
Physiological wound-healing progresses through three overlapping phases: inflammation, proliferation, and maturation.

The starting phase (inflammation) begins at the time of dermal damage, when the activation of the coagulation cascade causes release of cytokines that stimulate chemotaxis of neutrophils and macrophages into the wound.

After 48 to 72 hours, the healing process passes from the inflammation phase into the proliferation phase, which lasts 3 to 6 weeks. Fibroblasts are recruited into the wound in order to synthesize the scaffold of reparative tissue: the extracellular matrix (ECM). Granulation tissue is made by procollagen, elastin, proteoglycans, and hyaluronic acid. A particular population of fibroblasts called *myofibroblasts* that synthesize actin filaments are responsible for wound contraction.

Once the wound is healed, the immature scar passes into the final maturation phase, which may last a few months. ECM is progressively degraded and immature Type III collagen of early wound becomes finally mature Type I collagen.

The balance of synthesis and degradation of scar components shifts into a downregulation of healing, to allow the final scar to reach maximum organization and strength.

This multistep process is regulated by several molecules, including epidermal growth factor (EGF), basic fibroblast growth factor (bFGF), transforming growth factor-β (TGF-β), mitogen-activated protein kinases (MAPs), and metalloproteinases (MMPs).

Molecules that link these regulatory signals and the three phases of healing are only partially understood. In such a complicated system, vulnerabilities are not a remote possibility, which explains the relative facility of abnormal scar development in an inflammatory disease like acne.(2–5)

THE EVOLUTION OF INFLAMMATORY LESION TO SCAR DEVELOPMENT
Acne scar begins when noninflammatory comedone evolves into an inflammatory lesion that ruptures through the weakened infrainfundibular section of the follicle. Perifollicular abscess is the result of such a rupture. This will be repaired without scarring in 7 to 10 days. Cells grow from the epidermis and appendageal structures to circumscribe the inflammatory reaction. If this is complete, there is resolution of the lesion with no sequelae. Sometimes, however, the encapsulation is incomplete and further rupture occurs. The result may be the development of fistulous tracts. Clinical appearance consists of a group of open comedones with a number of interconnecting keratinized channels. Ice-pick scars represent an example of this evolution: Histopathological picture is characterized by reticulate tunnels lined by hyperplastic epithelium. Often there are remnants of inflammation even in old scars of this type.

Other types of outcome depend on the extent and depth of inflammation. When inflammation is deep, it will extend beyond the environment of the hair follicle into the subcutaneous tissue, along vascular channels and around sweat glands. The consequence is the destruction of subcutaneous fat and the development of deep scars.

ATROPHIC ACNE SCARS
In acne, atrophic scars are much more common than hypertrophic scars. They most commonly involve the dermis, but can also involve the underlying fat. The phases of healing include inflammation (in the infrainfundibular region of the pilosebaceous structure), granulation tissue formation with fibroplasia and neovascularization, wound contracture, and tissue remodelling.(6)

Enzymatic activity and inflammatory mediators also destroy the deeper structures.

Types of atrophic acne scars
The depth and the extent of inflammation will determine the degree of scar severity.

If only epidermis and superficial dermis are involved, scars may appear as macules that may be either erythematous or hyperchromic. This postinflammatory hyperpigmentation is more frequent, diffuse, and severe in patients with dark skin: With sunlight avoidance, its duration ranges between 3 months and 18 to 24 months. When middermis is involved, recurrent ruptures of follicles ensue and fistulae can occur. In such circumstances, excision of the entire pilosebaceous apparatus may be necessary.

If deep dermis is affected, sharp-walled or ice-pick scars are produced.

If more extensive dermal damage occurs, broad scars can develop, like rolling or boxcar scars.

At the trunk, follicular or perifollicular acne inflammation induces the development of hypopigmented scars.(7)

Hypertrophyc acne scars
In acne, the development of hypertrophic scars is uncommon.

In our clinical experience, these scars occur especially in male patients who suffered from severe varieties of papular-pustular or nodular acne, especially on the shoulders and back.

DIFFERENCES BETWEEN HYPERTROPHIC SCARS AND KELOIDS
The terms hypertrophic scar and keloid are often used interchangeably. Although there are some clinical similarities between hypertrophic scars and keloids, there are many biochemical, physiopathological, and clinical differences that support the fact that these entities are distinct.

Hypertrophic scars can appear everywhere; they are raised, with a smooth surface, pink to red in colour, and rarely accompanied by pruritus. Furthermore, hypertrophic scars do not extend beyond the margins of the original tissue damage. Hypertrophic scars evolve in a limited period of time: It is longer in comparison with normal scars, but its duration is less than a year.

Areas where keloids more frequently occur are the ears, upper portion of the chest, shoulders, arms, and the upper portion of the back. This suggests the existence of local populations of abnormal cells or tissue local factors that stimulate keloid development. The growth of keloids continues indefinitely, without a quiescent or regressive phase (8, 9); moreover, they extend to surrounding normal tissue, and pruritus is frequent. Some authors consider keloids a variety of benign fibrous tumour.

From the histopathological point of view, hypertrophic scars mainly contain Type III collagen: its fibers are thick and oriented parallel to the epidermal surface; furthermore, myofibroblasts are numerous Keloids are composed by disorganized Type I and III collagen bundles, with a low number of myofibroblasts. The collagen pattern is abnormally thick, with irregular branched septal collagen bands.(10–12) Both lesions demonstrate overproduction of multiple fibroblast proteins, suggesting either pathological persistence of healing signals or a failure of the appropriate downregulation of healing cells.(13, 14)

PATHOPHYSIOLOGY OF KELOIDS
The idea of a generic predisposition to keloid development has long been suggested; furthermore, affected patients often report a positive family history.(15, 16) A racial predisposition

in subjects with dark skin is well known. Keloids are usually observed in individuals between 10 and 30 years of age.(17)

Fibroblasts involved in keloid development are different, according to the phenotypical point of view, from those present in normal scars, and also if patients predisposed to keloid formation do not always develop abnormal scars.

Sometimes, after a normal initial evolution, some scars may become keloidal.(18) Keloid fibroblasts present an increased number of growth factor receptors and respond more quickly to growth factors, like platelet-derived growth factor (PDGF) and TGF-β that can upregulate these cells.(19) TGF-β is overproduced by keloid tissue and poorly regulated through normal signalling processes. A loss of feedback control during collagen and ECM production was demonstrated in keloid tissue.(20) Decreased synthesis of molecules that promote matrix breakdown and collagen organization may also explain the lack of scar regression observed in keloids. Abnormal epithelial–mesenchymal interactions, persistence of fetal wound–healing pathways, altered immune functions, failure of apoptosis, tissue hypoxia, and oxygen-free radical generation have also been suggested as causal factors of keloid growth.(21, 22)

REFERENCES
1. Layton AM, Henderson CA, Cunliffe WJ. A clinical evaluation of acne scarring and its incidence. Clin Exp Dermatol 1994; 19: 303–8.
2. Niessen FB, Spauwen PH, Schalkwijk J, Kon M. On the nature of hypertrophic scars and keloids: a review. Plast Reconstr Surg 1999; 104: 1435–58.
3. Pearson G, Robinson F, Beers Gibson T et al. Mitogen-activated protein (MAP) kinase pathways: regulation and physiological functions. Endocr Rev 2001; 22: 153–83.
4. Fujiwara M, Muragaki Y, Ooshima A. Keloid-derived fibroblasts show increased secretion of factors involved in collagen turnover and depend on matrix metalloproteinase for migration. Br J Dermatol 2005; 153: 295–300.
5. Tsujita-Kyutoku M, Uehara N, Matsuoka Y et al. Comparison of transforming growth factor-beta/Smad signaling between normal dermal fibroblasts and fibroblasts derived from central and peripheral areas of keloid lesions. In Vivo 2005; 19: 959–63.
6. Knutson DD. Ultrastructural observations in acne vulgaris: the normal sebaceous follicle and acne lesions. J Invest Dermatol 1974; 62: 288–307.
7. Wilson BB, Dent CH, Cooper PH. Papular acne scars. A common cutaneous finding. Arch Dermatol 1990; 126: 797–800.
8. Su CW, Alizadeh K, Boddie A, Lee RC. The problem scar. Clin Plast Surg 1998; 25: 451–65.
9. Burd A, Huang L. Hypertrophic response and keloid diathesis: two very different forms of scar. Plast Reconstr Surg 2005; 116: 150e–7e.
10. Editorial. Elastic tissue and hypertrophic scars. Burns 1976; 3: 407.

11. Ehrlich HP, Desmoulière A, Diegelmann RF et al. Morphological and immunochemical differences between keloid and hypertrophic scar. Am J Pathol 1994; 145: 105–13.
12. Blackburn WR, Cosman B. Histologic basis of keloid and hypertrophic scar differentiation. Clinicopathologic correlation. Arch Pathol 1966; 82: 65–71.
13. Younai S, Nichter LS, Wellisz T et al. Modulation of collagen synthesis by transforming growth factor-beta in keloid and hypertrophic scar fibroblasts. Ann Plast Surg 1994; 33: 148–51.
14. Bettinger DA, Yager DR, Diegelmann RF, Cohen IK. The effect of TGF-beta on keloid fibroblast proliferation and collagen synthesis. Plast Reconstr Surg 1996; 98: 827–33.
15. Bayat A, Walter JM, Bock O et al. Genetic susceptibility to keloid disease: mutation screening of the TGFbeta3 gene. Br J Plast Surg 2005; 58: 914–21.
16. Bayat A, Arscott G, Ollier WE, McGrouther DA, Ferguson MW. Keloid disease: clinical relevance of single versus multiple site scars. Br J Plast Surg 2005; 58: 28–37.
17. Lane JE, Waller JL, Davis LS. Relationship between age of ear piercing and keloid formation. Pediatrics 2005; 115: 1312–4.
18. Muir IF. On the nature of keloid and hypertrophic scars. Br J Plast Surg 1990; 43: 61–9.
19. Haisa M, Okochi H, Grotendorst GR. Elevated levels of PDGF alpha receptors in keloid fibroblasts contribute to an enhanced response to PDGF. J Invest Dermatol 1994; 103: 560–3.
20. Diegelmann RF, Cohen IK, McCoy BJ. Growth kinetics and collagen synthesis of normal skin, normal scar and keloid fibroblasts in vitro. J Cell Physiol 1979; 98: 341–6.
21. Kazeem AA. The immunological aspects of keloid tumor formation. J Surg Oncol 1988; 38: 16–8.
22. Cobbold CA. The role of nitric oxide in the formation of keloid and hypertrophic lesions. Med Hypotheses 2001; 57: 497–502.

3 Hypertrophic and keloidal scars
Maria Miteva and Paolo Romanelli

ACNE SCARS—GENERAL NOTES

The Merriam Webster's dictionary defines the word scar as "a mark left on the skin or other tissue after a wound, burn, pustule, lesion has healed; cicatrix." However, additional meanings stand for "a marring or disfiguring mark" as well as for "lasting mental or emotional effects of suffering or anguish." According to Koo et al., the psychological effects due to acne and acne scarring may lead to emotional debilitation, embarrassment, poor self-esteem, frustration, and social isolation.(1) Although these effects are difficult to quantify in patient terms, scarring that results from tissue damage and inflammation is a significant issue that requires attention and will be expanded herein with main focus on hypertrophic and keloidal scars (HS, KS).

Epidermal damage *per se* results in transient erythema and/or pigmentary disturbances such as postinflammatory hyperpigmentation, whereas dermal damage is more long lasting and accounts for decrease and increase of tissue. Tissue damage from acne inflammation can lead to permanent skin-texture changes and fibrosis, thus resulting in scar formation. Scars normally proceed through the specific phases of the wound-healing cascade: inflammation, granulation, and remodeling. However, even normal scars that have accomplished the healing process successfully achieve only 80% of previous skin strength.(2) Substantial amount of molecular and cellular data have been generated in an effort to understand the process of wound contraction and scar contracture formation. Basically, after completing the inflammatory and granulation phases, wound closure requires generation of proper contractile forces to close the wound. It has been shown that myofibroblasts appear to be intrinsically linked to the development of hypertrophic scars.(3) Migration of fibroblasts into and through the extracellular matrix during the initial phase of wound healing is a fundamental component of wound contraction. During this migration, the pulling of collagen fibrils into a streamlined pattern, and the associated production of collagenase, may facilitate a more normal arrangement of collagen. Once the wound has been repopulated and the chemotactic gradient that has been established by inflammatory cells is decreased, fibroblast migration will cease. It is at this point that myofibroblasts appear and play a key role in the production of hypertrophic scars.(3) Hence, one of the pivotal differences between wounds that proceed to normal scar (compared with those that develop hypertrophic scars) and scar contractures may be the lack and/or late induction of myofibroblast apoptotic cell death (see below for further details). The combined contribution of fibroblasts and myofibroblasts to abnormal extracellular matrix protein production results in an excessive and rigid scar. The isometric application of contractile forces by myofibroblasts probably contributes further to the formation of the whorls, nodules, and scar contractures characteristic of hypertrophic scars.

Acne scarring is a consequence of the damage that occurs in and around the pilosebaceous follicle during inflammation. However, the precise mechanisms and factors that govern the initiation and exacerbation of inflammation are not fully known. In a study of 185 patients with severe-grade acne on the face, chest, and back, Layton et al. showed that 95% of both sexes developed facial scarring to some degree.(4) The truncal region of male patients revealed significantly more total HS and KS than the same area of female patients. In this study HS and KS were most commonly seen in males and 85% of the patients affected had been previously noted to have nodular acne, and in the remaining 15%, only superficial inflammatory lesions had been appreciated. The sites of KS formation, in agreement with previous observations, were more commonly involving the back, shoulder, and chest, as well as the angle of the jaw. Furthermore, untreated acne lesions up to 3 years between initial onset and sufficient treatment regardless of sex or location were an important factor in determining resultant scarring. After this period, the degree of scarring did not increase significantly; the reason for that is still obscure.

Evidence suggests that acne is not a homogenous disease and that patients may generate different type of immune response since both Th1 and Th2 cytokine profiles have been found in established inflamed lesions from acne patients. Whether this difference contributes to the predisposition of some patients to scar was investigated in a study done by Holland et al.(5) Immunohistochemical methods were used to determine the cell-mediated immune response in developing and resolving inflamed lesions by examining the prevalence and activation states of lymphocyte subsets, macrophages, and endothelial cells, the major components of this response, present in two groups of patients with the same degree of inflamed acne but differing in their propensity to scar. The authors found out that the cellular infiltrate was large and active with a greater non-specific response (few memory T cells) and subsided in resolution in early lesions of patients who were not prone to scarring (NS). In contrast, a predominantly specific immune response was present in prone to scarring (S) patients—the infiltrate was initially smaller and ineffective, but the number of CD4+ T cells in the infiltrate remained increased and activated in resolving lesions. In addition, significant levels of angiogenesis also persisted, thus facilitating a prolonged inflammatory response. However, the majority of CD4+ T cells were skin-homing memory effector cells, with the absence of unclassified cells, suggesting that S patients are more susceptible to the causative antigens. The authors concluded that in S patients there is a

11

chronic, delayed-type hypersensitivity reaction provoked by a persistent antigenic stimulus that these patients are probably unable to eliminate initially.

Furthermore, in a recently published study, significant differences were observed in the expression levels of members of caspase, cytokines, and MAP-kinase pathways, between the normal skin of keloid-prone and keloid-resistant patients. Specifically, expression of caspase 6, and caspase 14 genes were different between normal skin of keloid-prone individuals and keloid-resistant patients. These results suggest that normal skin of keloid-prone individuals constitutively expresses a distinct gene profile that might contribute to their susceptibility to develop keloids.(6)

There are two principal causes of acne scar formation: either as a result of loss/damage of tissue or less common due to increased tissue formation. The first category comprises three primary types of acne scars as described by Jacob et al.(7): icepick, rolling, and boxcar, commonly seen on the cheeks. Treatment is frequently done by punch excision with closure, resurfacing or punch elevation, as well as by subcision. Nevertheless, this category of scars is out of the scope of our chapter and, therefore, will not be discussed further.

Objective evaluation of acne scars is controversial since most of the grading approaches are not applicable in practical, daily use by the average physician.(8) There are grading devices that focus on 3-dimensional grid-based mapping of lesions and molded skin replicas for comparison examination.(9) However, some grading scales for acne scars are more practical for day-to-day implementation. In 1999, the ECLA (echelle d'evaluation clinique des lesions d'acne) was introduced (10), followed by the ECCA (echelle d'evaluation clinique des cicatrices d'acne) (11) in 2006. Using this scale, the qualitative aspects of scars define the type of scar, which is then associated with a quantitative score (0–4) determined semiquantitatively and multiplied by a weighting factor (15–50) of clinical severity, leading to possible totals of 0 to 540. It was found to have good interinvestigator reliability, although it did not focus on ice-pick-, rolling-, or boxcar-type scars specifically, but rather on variations of atrophic and hypertrophic scars. Goodman and Baron (12) described another quantitative grading system based on counting (1–10, 11–20, > 20) of scar type (atrophic, macular, boxcar, hypertrophic, keloidal) and severity (mild, moderate, severe). Points are assigned to each respective category and totaled within the range of a minimum of 0 to a maximum of 84. The same physicians also outlined a qualitative (rather than quantitative) grading system (13) that is simpler for quick, daily use. It distinguished four grades for level of disease: (1) macular, (2) mild, (3) moderate, and (4) severe. Subdivisions of macular disease are erythematous, hyperpigmented, or hypopigmented, and those of mild to severe disease are atrophic and hypertrophic. Further specification includes the number of cosmetic units involved: "A" for focal or one lesion and "B" for discrete or two to three lesions. In conclusion, all these systems and variations can become quite confusing. Moreover, the lack of a true consensus scale hinders standardization of diagnosis and treatment of acne scarring.

We will focus on the second group of scars that result from excess tissue formation in patients with acne vulgaris, that is, HS and KS. Initially, the epidemiology, clinical characteristics, and pathogenesis of HS and KS are covered and then several of treatment options currently available are discussed.

DEFINITION AND CLINICAL CHARACTERISTICS OF HS AND KS

HS and KS are two patterns of benign fibrous growths that show abnormal wound-healing responses in predisposed individuals (**Figure 3.1A,B**). They result from an exaggerated connective tissue response to trauma, inflammation, surgery, or burns, and occasionally seem to occur spontaneously.(14) Whether a skin injury would lead to a HS or a KS depends on the duration of the fibroblast exposure to microenvironmental influences that alter the cellular and molecular processes that foster increased collagen production.(15, 16) *HS* are characterized by

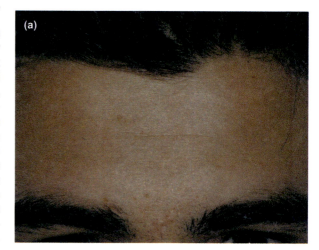

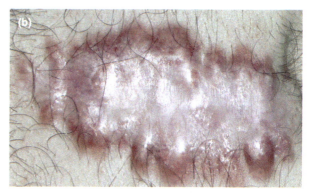

Figure 3.1 (A) Hypertrophic scars in a patient with acne vulgaris—clinical presentation. (B) Keloidal scar in a patient with acne vulgaris—clinical presentation.

Table 3.1 Juxtaposition of clinical and molecular features.

Hypertrophic Scars	Keloidal Scars
Develop soon after surgery	Many develop months after injury/surgery
Usually subside with time	Rarely subside with time
Limited within wound boundaries	Overgrow wound boundaries
Size correlates with injury surface	Minor injury may produce larger lesions
Occur with motion	Independent of motion
May induce contractures over joints	Do not induce contractures
Improve after appropriate surgery	Often worsens after surgery
Collagen bundles are fine, well organized, wavy parallel to epidermis	Collagen bundles are large, thick, closely packed, random to epidermis
Myofibroblasts present	Devoid of myofibroblasts
SMA expression—nodular, diffuse	SMA expression—around blood vessels
Negative for mucin	Focal expression for mucin in the dermis
Apoptosis—decreased	Apoptosis—increased
Low p53	High p53

elevation above the skin surface, redness, and itching. They are limited to the borders of the injury, tend to regress with time, are susceptible to plastic surgery revision, and may produce scar contractures when located over joints.(17) Scars that cross joints or skin creases at right angles are especially likely to form HS, possibly because of the constant tension forces that occur. Initial lesions are often erythematous, become brownish-red, and then pale as they age. They are usually void of hair follicles and other functioning adnexal glands. HS rarely elevate more than 4 mm above the skin surface.

KS are also red and itchy, but they exceed the boundaries of the initial injury, do not regress with time, are difficult to revise surgically, and do not provoke contractures. KS may follow trauma, sometimes with delay of months. However, spontaneous KS have been known to develop (especially on the midchest area) in patients who deny any preceding trauma. (18) Certain body regions show increased susceptibility to keloids. The deltoid, presternal, and upper-back regions, and earlobes seem to be most commonly affected. KS formation in the eyelids, genitalia, palms, or soles is unusual.(17) KS range in size from papules a few millimeters in diameter to ball size or larger. Those on the ears, neck, and abdomen tend to be pedunculated, whereas those on the central chest, upper back, and extremities are usually raised with a flat surface with the base being wider than the top. KS range in consistency from soft and doughy to rubbery hard. They project usually more than 4 mm above the level of the surrounding skin but rarely extend into the underlying subcutaneous tissue (19–21) (Table 3.1).

NEW INSIGHTS INTO THE MOLECULAR BIOLOGY OF HYPERTROPHIC SCARS AND KELOIDS

There are several excellent reviews discussing extensively the molecular an cellular pathology of HS and KS (14, 15, 21, 22). Herein, we would briefly refer to a few of the most current directions in HS and KS research regarding the fibrogenic response

to trauma as a function of Th1/Th2 interplay, Transforming growth factor-β (TGF-β) as a target for new scar treatment approach, scar extracellular matrix (ECM) remodeling, and apoptosis and differentiation of fibrogenic cells.

Collagen synthesis in KS is approximately 20 times greater than in normal unscarred skin and 3 times greater than in hypertrophic scars.(14) Apart from the foregoing discussion on the concept of abnormal wound healing due to longer persistence of fibroblasts in HS and KS than in normal scar tissue (in which they would regress after the third week) (23), there is another related concept that puts forward the possibility that the amount of fibrosis is not necessarily linked to the severity of inflammation.(24–27) The recruitment of T lymphocytes, specifically CD4+ T helper cells, to the early wound has been the focus of recent interest. The characteristic cytokine expression profile of the CD4+ T cells is the basis for describing either a predominantly Th1 or Th2 response to a stimulus. The development of a Th2 response (with production of IL-4, IL-5, IL-10, and IL-13) has been strongly linked to fibrogenesis. IL-4 is considered to be nearly twice as potent at mediating fibrosis as TGF-β. Although an equally strong inflammatory response develops with a predominance of Th1, CD4+ cells, which produce interferon IFN-γ and IL-12, the development of tissue fibrosis is almost completely attenuated.(28) A further study into the mechanisms of Th1 cell-mediated antifibrotic effects has revealed expression of acute-phase reaction and proapoptotic genes by these T cells. Furthermore, Th1 cytokines activate nitric oxide synthase (NOS) expression that promotes collagenase activity and matrix remodeling. This may explain the large degree of cell apoptosis and matrix digestion observed when a polarized Th1 cell response is prolonged. Fibroblasts from HS and KS exhibit reduced collagenase activity in combination with reduced nitric oxide (NO) production and NOS activity, suggesting that these fibroblasts are likely not subject to a Th1 response.

It is now known that growth factors play a role in contraction. TGF-β and platelet-derived growth factor (PDGF) have recently been shown to be key factors in modulating contraction in normal skin fibroblasts.(29) TGF-β strongly promotes the chemotaxis of fibroblasts to the site of inflammation to begin the production of extracellular matrix proteins. The activity of TGF-β is normally turned off when repair is complete. Dysregulation of TGF-β production or activity can cause abnormal fibrosis. Strong and persistent expression of TGF-b and its receptors has been shown in fibroblasts of postburn HS.(30) It has also been identified that the serum of recovering burn patients contains levels of TGF-β about twice as much as those in control patients.(31) Furthermore, the ontogenetic transition from scarless fetal wound healing to adult scarring is believed to be TGF-β dependent. TGF-β expression is only transiently expressed in scarless fetal wounds and to a much lesser amount than in adult wound healing. TGF-β receptors I and II are also expressed less.(32) Probably the most compelling evidence for a causative role of TGF-β in producing scar lies in the finding of scar formation in fetal wounds treated with TGF-β.(33)

Quantitative analysis of ECM components in scar samples has facilitated the understanding of some of the physical properties of abnormal scars. Elastic fibers are present in large amounts in normal skin, especially in youth. In pathological conditions such as fibrosis, elastic fibers may be present in even higher levels. The influence of elastin on contraction of ECM, however, is unknown. Using a stereological method for quantifying antibody staining of cross-sectional tissue sections, a decrease in fibrillin-1 and elastin density was found in HS versus normal skin.(26) Interestingly, the proportion of elastin was higher in the deep dermal layer of KS. The mechanism of these changes in microfibril composition remains poorly understood. (34) The major effectors of ECM degradation and remodeling belong to a family of structurally related enzymes called metaloproteinases (MMPs). MMPs are secreted in an inactive form requiring activation by means of proteolytic cleavage. During cutaneous wound repair, the activity of MMP-2 and MMP-9 persists after wound closure and seems to be important in the remodeling process.(35) In particular, HS and KS are found to have high levels of MMP-2 and low levels of MMP-9. MMP-2 plays a major role in matrix remodeling later in wound healing, degrading denatured collagen. MMP-9 is typically involved in early wound repair and can degrade native Type IV and V collagen, elastin, fibronectin, and denatured collagen of all types.(36) Keloid fibroblasts show a 2.5-fold increase in migratory activity compared with normal dermal fibroblasts, which is associated with increased production of type I collagen, MMP-1, MMP-2, and TIMP-1 by keloid fibroblasts. The acceleration of the remodeling process possibly through the enhancement of MMP activity may be a useful therapeutic approach for these scars.

Apoptosis, programmed cell death, is morphologically and biochemically distinct from other forms of cell death. Recently, apoptosis has been shown to participate in the transition between granulation tissue and the formation of scar after tissue injury.(37–40) The regulation of apoptosis during wound healing may thus be an important factor in normal and pathologic scarring. Normal cellular proliferation in skin is regulated by growth-promoting protooncogenes counterbalanced by growth-constraining tumor-suppressor genes and regulators of apoptosis such as the bcl-2 gene family.(41, 42) The p53 tumor-suppressor gene has been linked to apoptosis pathways via its effect on bcl-2 gene expression. Focal dysregulation of p53 combined with upregulation of bcl-2 may help produce a combination of increased cell proliferation and decreased cell death in younger keloids areas with high cell density.(40) Differences in apoptotic profiles between normal wound-healing myofibroblasts and HS myofibroblasts have been described.(37, 40) Normal wound-healing myofibroblasts are less resistant to apoptosis than dermal fibroblasts, whereas HS myofibroblasts are more resistant. Similarly, keloid fibroblasts have been shown to possess greater proliferative capacity than normal fibroblasts, and they are more resistant to apoptosis than normal dermal fibroblasts.(19, 40) p53 and p63 genes play distinct and overlapping roles in apoptosis and subsequently in scar formation and development of unfavorable scars. The expression of p53 seems to be related to scar maturation. It can be speculated that keloidal fibroblasts resist physiologic cell death and, therefore, continue to proliferate and produce collagen.(41–43)

In line with this and in order to clarify the importance of apoptosis in hypertrophic scar formation, a recent study has examined the effects of mechanical loading on cutaneous wounds of animals with altered pathways of cellular apoptosis.(44) In p53-null mice, with downregulated cellular apoptosis, the authors observed significantly greater scar hypertrophy and cellular density. Conversely, scar hypertrophy and cellular density are significantly reduced in proapoptotic bcl-2-null mice. They concluded that mechanical loading early in the proliferative phase of wound healing produces hypertrophic scars by inhibiting cellular apoptosis through an Akt-dependent mechanism (where Akt is a prosirvival marker).

HISTOLOGY OF HS AND KS

Morphological and immunohistochemical differences do exist between HS and KS. In KS abnormally large collagen-bundle complexes are identified, whereas these are absent in HS. These complex collagen bundles are shown to be associated with important amounts of "ground substance"—mucopolysaccharides. A histological characteristic of HS is the presence of nodules containing a high density of cells and collagen. They are cigar shaped and run parallel to the surface of the skin, are located in the middle or deeper layer of the scar, and are oriented along the tension lines of the scar. Fibroblasts in nodules have been reported to have long processes that are intimately attached to the collagen fibers. The absence of such nodules is a characteristic of a KS (Figure 3.2A,B).

However, it is sometimes difficult to differentiate between HS and KS on light microscopy solely. Making the correct diagnosis in ambiguous cases is important because this may be crucial for directing the right treatment. Ehrlich et al. investigated the

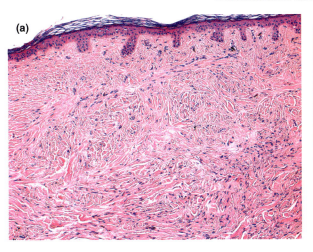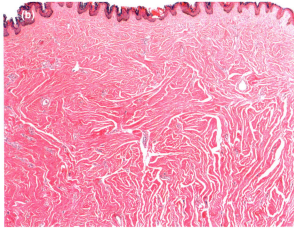

Figure 3.2 (A) Hypertrophic scar—histology, H&E 10X: collagen bundles are flatter, less demarcated and arranged in a wavy pattern. Most of the bundles lie parallel to the skin surface. Myofibroblasts are dispersed among collagen bundles. (B) Keloid—histology, H&E 4X: collagen bundles are basically nonexistent; they lie in haphazardly connected loose sheets which appear randomly oriented to the skin surface. Lesion appears homogenous and is devoid of myofibroblasts.

collagen organization and the possible presence of α-smooth muscle actin expressing myofibroblasts (SMA) in both conditions.(17) They were able to confirm that nodular structures are always present in HS, but rarely in KS. Furthermore, only nodules of HS contain SMA+ myofibroblasts. Electron microscopic examination supports the above-mentioned differences in collagen organization and in fibroblastic features and shows the presence of an amorphous extracelular material surrounding fibroblastic cells in KS. The presence in HS of myofibroblasts positive for the isoform of SMA typical of vascular smooth muscle cells may represent an important element in the pathogenesis of contraction. Interestingly, when placed in culture, fibroblasts from HS and KS express similar amounts of SMA, suggesting that local microenvironmental factors influence *in vivo* the expression of this protein.

HS AND KS TREATMENT

Numerous options for treatment of acne HS and KS have been available over the years with variable success. They are mainly divided into two big groups: surgical and nonsurgical treatments that can be utilized either as single-use or as combined modalities. However, definitive therapies remain elusive due to problems related to standardization of study designs.(21) In this chapter, we will cover briefly only a few of the most commonly used and/or evidence-supported approaches. More information on the use of other treatments such as retinoids, intralesional (IL) bleomycin, 5-fluorouracil, verapamil, intralesional hyaluronidase, and so on can be found elsewhere.(14, 45–47)

Silicone can be used to prevent HS formation as well as to treat developed scars. Several clinically controlled and randomized studies have confirmed the effectiveness of silicone-gel sheeting in HS and KS.(48, 49) However, not all clinical studies showed good results (50), possibly because treatment and control areas were adjacent, and also because of the possible overlapping of the silicone sheet or the immaturity of the scars. A recently published review on the biologic effects, clinical efficacy, and safety of silicone elastomer sheeting for HS and KS treatment (51) concluded that silicone elastomer sheeting appears to be an effective option for treating and preventing HS with minimal side effects. Furthermore, it could be used in combination with other modalities and is easy to access. Clinicians recommend that the silicone elastomer sheeting be in contact with the HS for 12 to 24 hours per day for 6 to 12 months, with removal permitted for routine hygiene and/or when temporary adverse effects such as pruritus, miliaria rash, and maceration occur. Finally, a recently published study showed a better effect of silicone gel over silicone elastomer sheeting in regards to scar elevation improvement in HS.(52)

Pressure therapy. At present, pressure therapy is a preferred method for conservative management of scars, especially in hypertrophic burn scars, to increase thinning and improve pliability of the scars.(53) However, clinical effectiveness has never been scientifically proven.(46) Treatment is most effective if the HS is still active; therefore, less improvement is expected after 6 months.(54) It is recommended that a garment is worn for 18 to 24 hours a day with a pressure between 24 and 40 mmHg until the scar matures. Unfortunately, premature release of the garment may lead to rebound hypertrophy.(20)

Intralesional steroids (IL GKS). One of the most popular choices for medical therapy of HS and KS is the use of the generically termed "steroids." These are substances based on four fused carbon rings that derive from the cholesterol molecule. The glucocorticoids (e.g., triamcinolone, hydrocortisone, methylprednisone, and dexamethasone), in the corticosteroid family, have immunomodulatory and antiinflammatory properties.(8) The exact mechanism of action in HS and KS is unknown, but it is thought to be related directly to the antiinflammatory properties, reduction of collagen, glycosaminoglycans, and fibroblasts, along with overall lesion growth retardation. There are several routes of administration: topical, both with and without occlusion, as intralesional injections, and in the setting of combination approaches such as IL GKS and silicone gel sheeting.(47) However, topical application is associated with questionable rate of absorption. Hence, the IL administration of GKS is often the preferred choice in the practice. Steroids, most commonly triamcinolone acetonide 10–40 mg/ml, can be injected IL at 4-to-6-week intervals .The maximum dose is 1 mg (= 0.1ml of 10 mg/ml) per injection with at least 1 cm gap between injection sites. The maximum amount of injections is not known, although, according to some (46), the total dosage should not exceed 30 to 40 mg; this means the maximum treatable scar surface is approximately 40 cm^2. Therefore, one should realize that this therapy is not suitable for extensive scars.(46, 55) Further disadvantages of this approach include side effects such as telangiectases, bruising, atrophy, pain, or pigmentary changes.

Surgical management is an essential tool in the treatment of ice-pick, rolling, and boxcar scars. However, in regards to HS and KS, surgical intervention must be done with care because such patients are known to have propensity for such a response. If undertaken, some recommend that the incision is done within the lesion boundaries to prevent further extension and that the effect is closed primarily. In addition, steroids are commonly administered locally.(8) Therefore, the goal would be more to reduce overall size or debulk rather than completely excise. Secondary, refining procedures may also be used in the areas if desired or needed. In a study of 21 patients (10 males, 11 females; age 17–59 years, mean age 35.52 years; Fitzpatrick skin type I-III) there was good improvement, as rated by both independent assessors and patients, when laser resurfacing was done after punch excision of scars.(56) This approach has an advantage in that punch excision eliminates the deeper components and allows for only superficial laser treatment with fewer passes. Finally, if surgery is done, postoperative laser resurfacing may also come into consideration because the chance of unwanted side effects could thus be reduced.

Cryotherapy can be used either as a monotherapy for HS and KS or in combination with other modalities such as IL GKS. The primary object of cryotherapy is to induce ischemic damage of the microcirculation. As a result, the cellular destruction and anoxia promotes shrinkage of the hypertrophic scar tissue. A tendency to normalization of the collagen structure after treatment in HS and KS suggests recovery of normal collagen synthesis. One study reported over 50% scar volume reduction after one intralesional treatment in

HS and KS, without recurrence during 18 months of follow-up.(57) Younger KS and HS seem to respond better to cryosurgery than the older ones do.(58) When compared to IL GKS, cryosurgery was found to be significantly better for early vascular lesions of less than 12-month's duration.(59) The pain caused by application of liquid nitrogen, although generally not severe, is a drawback for some patients, especially when the keloid to be treated is fairly large. A certain degree of atrophy and hypopigmentation is also inevitable with this approach, thus making it less preferable for lesions located on the face and upper chest. Furthermore, this characteristic feature would probably render cryosurgery less applicable in dark-skinned patients.(58)

Radiation for the treatment of HS has not been described frequently, in contrast to the application in KS in which especially brachytherapy is successful. Most likely, this is due to lack of efficacy in HS and serious adverse effects, such as hyperpigmentation, pruritus and erythema, and rarely, even poikiloderma. Radiation use is derived from the destruction of fibroblast vasculature, decrease of fibroblast activity, and local cellular apoptosis. It has been found that the regrowth of keloids is proportional to the total dose of irradiation given and that 900 cGy is the minimal effective dose recommended. Initiation of treatment, size of the largest fraction given, fractionation of doses, duration of treatment, or location of lesion are less important. This modality is used more as an adjunct to prevent a recurrence rather than a stand-alone treatment. A Japanese study involving 38 patients with keloids (ear, neck, and upper lip) who were treated with surgical excision and postoperative irradiation on average day 4.0 ± 4.9, with follow-up at a mean of 4.4 ± 2.5 years, showed significant improvement of pigmentation, pliability, height, vascularity, and hardness. Recurrence rate was 21.2% overall with none observed in the craniofacial area. Thus, it was concluded that surgical excision plus electron beam radiation started within a few days is beneficial in both controlling scar quality and preventing recurrence.(60)

Laser and light therapy. In scar management, the use of lasers has gained significance. With the use of first carbon dioxide and argon lasers in the treatment of HS, recurrence rates of 90% and higher were seen.(43, 47) In combination with IL GKS outcomes improved, although recurrence rates remained high at 16% to 74%.(61) It is currently accepted that the optimal nonablative laser to use for HS and KS is the 585-nm pulsed-dye laser (PDL). Best results and least side effects are obtained on Fitzpatrick skin types I or II because of decreased competition with melanin.(62, 63) This laser focuses on erythema and vascularity; therefore, incidental scar improvement is possibly due to decreasing vascularity. Its secondary effects refer to other cellular alterations, specifically collagen architecture. Improvement after use can be seen up to a year later. One study involving 15 patients with erythematous, hypertrophic scars treated with 510- or 585-nm PDL, with the objective of observing pigmentation and/or erythema improvement, found incidental improvement in scar texture and elevation. This was most likely a result from decreased perfusion and nutrition with resultant anoxia, cell death, and enzymatic changes.(64) In another study, an optical profilometry was used to evaluate the 585-nm PDL effect on previously argon laser–treated port wine stains. It was found that there was improvement of hypertrophic and atrophic scar regions as exhibited by flattening and reappearance of skin markings, respectively. The authors concluded that a part of the improvement may be attributed to eradication of enlarged blood vessels trapped within the sclerotic collagen.(65)

The 1064-nm neodymium:YAG (Nd:YAG) laser has demonstrated effects similar to those discussed for PDLs in regards to HS and KS. One small observational study using short-pulsed 1064-nm Nd:YAG lasers showed improvement in 100% of subjects' scars. Self-assessment done by the patients revealed that they were all satisfied with the results and would undergo the same treatment again.(66)

NEW THERAPEUTIC DEVELOPMENTS

Interferon—Interferons (INF) are naturally occurring antifibrotic cytokines that are reported to have beneficial therapeutical effect in abnormal scars because they cause a decrease of the synthesis of collagen type I and III by fibroblasts and an increase in collagenase activity.(67) Biopsies of hypertrophic burn scars treated with systemic INFα-2b showed a decreased number of fibroblasts compared with biopsies of immature burn scars and normotrophic scars.(68, 69) A reduction in serum TGF-β concentration could also play a role in scar reduction. It was suggested that improvement of hypertrophic scars after injection is associated with induction of myofibroblast apoptosis. Tredget et al. have shown significant improvement of hypertrophic burn scars in 78% of the patients after interferon therapy.(31) Adverse effects of interferon therapy include flu-like symptoms and pain on injection site.

Onion extract/heparin gel is another field of current research interest. It has been used in the treatment of HS.(70, 71) In a comparative study of 107 patients, Ho et al. showed that scar development after surgery was less in onion extract—or heparin gel–treated scars than in untreated scars.(71) The onion extract possesses fibroblast-inhibiting properties that reduce fibroproliferative activity and the production of the extracellular matrix. Heparin may also play an important role as it interacts with collagen molecules. However, heparin will also have systemic effects.

Other current research options include studying the effect of substances derived from plants that have antiinflammatory properties. Most of them have previously shown antitumor effect and are now explored for their properties to inhibit keloid fibroblast proliferation too. One such substance is quercetin, a common flavonoid in medical plants. More information about this and other "immunonutrition" derivates as well as fatty acid therapeutic agents can be found elsewhere.(15, 72–75)

In conclusion scarring is a common complication of acne vulgaris in the general population, particularly in individuals of color

and/or males. There are multiple options that can be tailored to each individual's needs, tolerance, and expectations along with the physician's assessments, skills, and preferences. Intralesional steroids are the mainstay of treatment. Modern options include laser or energy-derived therapies that need further verification for efficacy and safety. Currently, the utmost goal is significant improvement rather than complete clearance of the acne scars.

REFERENCES

1. Koo J. The psychosocial impact of acne: patients' perceptions. J Am Acad Dermatol 1995; 32(Suppl): S26–30.
2. Rivera AE. Clinical aspects of full-thickness wound healing. Clin Dermatol 2007; 25: 39–48.
3. Nedelec B, Ghahary A, Scott PG, Tredget EE. Control of wound contraction. Basic and clinical features. Hand Clin 2000; 16(2): 289–302.
4. Layton AM, Handerson CA, Cunliffe WJ. A clinical evaluation of acne scarring and its incidence. Clin Exp Dermatol 1994; 19: 303–8.
5. Holland DB, Jeremy AHT, Roberts SG et al. Inflammation in acne scarring: a comparison of the responses in lesions from patients prone and not prone to scar. Br J Dermatol 2004; 150: 72–81.
6. Nassiri M. Woolery-Lloyd H, Ramos S et al. Gene expression profiling reveals alteration of caspase 6 and 14 transcripts in normal skin of keloid-prone patients. Arch Dermatol Res 2008; in press.
7. Jacob CI, Dover JS, Kainer MS. Acne scarring: a classification and review of treatment options. J Am Acad Dermatol 2001; 45: 109–17.
8. Rivera AE. Acne scarring: a review and current treatment modalities. J Am Acad Dermatol 2008; 59: 659–76.
9. Friedman PM, Skover GR, Payonk G., Kauvar ANB, Geronemus, RG. 3D in-vivo optical skin imaging for topographical quantitative assessment of non-ablative laser technology. Dermatol Surg 2002; 28: 199–204.
10. Dreno B, Bodokh I, Chivot M et al. ECLA grading: a system of acne classification for every day dermatological practice. Ann Dermatol Venereol 1999; 126: 136–41.
11. Dreno B, Khammari A, Orain N et al. ECCA grading scale: an original validated acne scar grading scale for clinical practice in dermatology. Dermatology 2007; 214: 46–51.
12. Goodman GJ, Baron JA. Postacne scarring–a quantitative global scarring grading system. J Cosmet Dermatol 2006; 5: 48–52.
13. Goodman G, Baron JA. Post acne scarring–a qualitative global scarring grading system. Dermatol Surg 2006; 32: 1458–66.
14. English RS, Shenefelt PD. Keloids and hypertrophic scars. Dermatol Surg 1999; 25: 631–8.
15. Louw L. The keloid phenomenon: progress toward a solution. Clin Anat 2007; 20: 3–14.
16. Alster TS, Tanzi EL. Hypertrophic scars and keloids. Am J Clin Dermatol 2003; 4: 235–43.

17. Ehrlich PH, Desmouliere A, Diegelmann RF et al. Morphological and immunochemical differences between keloid and hypertrophic scar. Am J Pathol 1994; 145: 105–13.

18. Murray JC. Scars and keloids. Dermatol Clin 1993; 11: 697–707.

19. Koese O, Waseem A. Keloids and hypertrophic scars: are they two different sides of the same coin? Dermatol Surg 2008; 34: 336–46.

20. Niessem FP, Spawen HM, Schakwjk J et al. On the nature of hypertrophic scars and keloids: a review. Plast Reconstr Surg 1999; 104: 1435–58.

21. Shaffer RS, Shenefelt PD. Keloids and hypertrophic scars: a review with a critical look at therapeutic options. J Am Acad Dermatol 2002; 46: S63–97.

22. Datuba-Brown DD. Keloids: a review of the literature. Br J Plast Surg 1990; 43: 70–7.

23. Nakaoka H, Miyachi S, Miki Y. Proliferating activity of dermal fibroblastsin keloids and hypertrophic scars. Acta Derm Venereol (Stockh) 1995; 75: 102–4.

24. Wynn T. Fibrotic disease and the TH1/TH2 paradigm. Nature Rev Immunol 2004; 4: 583–94.

25. Doucet C, Brouty-Boye D, Pottin-Clemenceau C et al. IL-4 and IL-13 act on human lung fibroblasts. J Clin Invest 1998; 101: 2129–39.

26. Armour A, Scott PG, Tredget EE. Cellular and molecular pathology of HTS: basis for treatment. Wound Rep Reg 2007; 15: S6–17.

27. Gordon S. Alternative activation of macrophages. Nature Rev Immunol 2003; 3: 23–5.

28. Hoffmann KF, Cheever AW, Wynn TA. IL-10 and the dangers of immune polarization: excessive type 1 and type 2 cytokine responses induce distinct forms of lethal immunopathology in murine schistosomiasis. J Immunol 2000; 164: 6406–16.

29. Jagadeesan J, Bayat A. Transforming growth factor beta (TGF b) and kelod disease. Int J Surg 2007; 5: 278–85.

30. Lee T, Chin G, Kim W et al. Expression of transforming growth factor beta 1, 2 and 3 proteins in keloids. Ann Plast Surg 1999; 43: 179–84.

31. Tredget E, Shankowsky H, Pannu R et al. Transforming growth factor beta in thermally injured patients with hypertrophic scars:effects of interferon alpha-2b. Plast Reconstr Surg 1998; 102: 1317–28.

32. Chen W, Fu X, Ge S et al. Ontogeny of expression of transforming growth factor-beta and its receptors and their possible relationship with scarless healing in human fetal skin. Wound Repair Regen 2005; 13: 68–75.

33. Bock O, Yu H, Zitron S et al. Studies of transforming growth factors beta 1-3 and their receptors I and II in fibroblasts of keloid and hypertrophic scars. Acta Dermato-Venereol 2005; 85: 216–20.

34. Amadeu T, Braune A, Porto L, Desmouliere A, Costa A. Fibrillin-1 and elastin are differentially expressed in hypertrophic scars and keloids. Wound Repair Regen 2004; 12: 169–74.

35. Fujiwara M, Muragaki Y, Ooshima A. Keloid-derived fibroblasts show increased secretion of factors involved in collagen turnover and depend on matrix metalloproteinase for migration. Br J Dermatol 2005; 153: 295–300.

36. Zhang Y, McCluskey K, Fujii K, Wahl L. Differential regulation of monocyte matrix metalloproteinase and TIMP-1 production by TNF-alpha, granulocyte-macrophage CSF and IL-1beta through prostaglandin-dependent and independent mechanisms. J Immunol 1998; 61: 3071–6.

37. Teofoli P, Barduagni S, Ribuffo M et al. Expression of Bcl-2, p53, c-jun and c-fos protooncogenes in keloids and hypertrophic scars. J Dermatol Sci 1999; 22: 31–7.

38. Akasaka Y, Fujita K, Ishikawa Y et al. Detection of apoptosis in keloids and a comparative study on apoptosis between keloids, hypertrophic scars, normal healed flat scars, and dermatofibroma. Wound Rep Regen 2001; 9: 501–6.

39. Moulin V, Larochelle S, Langlois C et al. Normal skin wound and hypertrophic scar myofibroblasts have differential responses to apoptotic inductors. J Cell Physiol 2004; 198: 350–8.

40. Tanaka A, Hatoko M, Tada H et al. Expression of p53 family in scars. J Dermatol Sci 2004 34: 17–24.

41. Desmouliere A, Redard M, Darby I et al. Apoptosis mediates the decrease in cellularity during the transition between granulation tissue and scar. Am J Pathol 1995; 146: 56–66.

42. Moulin V, Larochelle S, Langlois C et al. Normal skin wound and hypertrophic scar myofibroblasts have differential responses to apoptotic inductors. J Cell Physiol 2004; 198: 350–8.

43. Niessen FB, Scalkwjk J, Vos H et al. Hypertrophic scar formation is associated with an increased number of epidermal Langerhans cells. J Pathol 2004; 20: 121–9.

44. Aarabi S, Bhatt KA, Shi Y et al. Mechanical load initiates hypertrophic scar formation through decreased cellular apoptosis. FASEB J 2007; 21: 3250–61.

45. Tsau SS, Dover JS, Arndt KA, Kaminer MS. Scar management: keloid, hypertrophic, atrophic and acne scars. Semin Cutan Med Surg 2002; 21: 46–75.

46. Bloemen MC, van der Veer WM, Ulrich MM et al. Prevention and curative management of hypertrophic scar formation. Burns 2008; in press.

47. Mustoe TA, Cooter RD, Gold MH et al. International clinical recommendations on scar management. Plast Reconstr Surg 2002; 110: 560–71.

48. Li-Tsang CW, Lau JC, Chan CC. Prevalence of hypertrophic scar formation and its characteristics among the Chinese population. Burns 2005; 31: 610–6.

49. Ahn ST, Monafo WW, Mustoe TA. Topical silicone gel: a new treatment for hypertrophic scars. Surgery 1989; 106: 781–6.

50. Wittenberg GP, Fabian BG, Bogomilsky JL et al. Prospective, single-blind, controlled study to assess the efficacy of the 585-nm flashlamp-pumped pulsed-dye laser and silicone and g.s.i.h.s. treatment., Arch Dermatol Clin 1999; 135: 1049–55.

51. Berman B, Perez OA, Konda S et al. A review on the biologic effects, clinical efficacy, and safety of silicone elastomer sheeting for hypertrophic scars and keloid scar treatment and management. Dermatol Surg 2007; 33: 1291–303.
52. Chernoff WG, Cramer H, Su-Huang S. The efficacy of topical silicone gel elastomers in the treatment of hypertrophic scars, keloid scars, and post-laser exfoliation erythema. Aesthetic Plast Surg 2007; 31: 495–500.
53. Reno F, Grazianetti P, Cannas M. Effects of mechanical compression on hypertrophic scars: prostaglandin E2 release. Burns 2001; 27: 215–8.
54. Zurada JM, Kriegel D, Davis IC. Topical treatments for hypertrophic scars. J Am Acad Dermatol 2006; 55: 1024–31.
55. Brissett AE, Sherris DA. Scar contractures, hypertrophic scars, and keloids. Facial Plast Surg 2001; 17: 263–72.
56. Grevelink JM, White VR. Concurrent use of laser skin resurfacing and punch excision in the treatment of facial acne scarring. Dermatol Surg 1998; 24: 527–30.
57. Har-Shai Y, Amar M, Sabo E. Intralesional cryotherapy for enhancing the involution of hypertrophic scars and keloids. Plast Reconstr Surg 2003; 111: 1841–52.
58. Rusciani L, Rossi G, Bono R. Use of cryotherapy in the treatment of keloids. J Dermatol Surg Oncol 1993; 19: 529–34.
59. Rockwell WB, Cohen IK, Ehrlich HP. Keloids and hypertrophic scars. A comprehensive review. Plast Reconstr Surg 1989; 84: 827–37.
60. Akita S, Akino K, Yakabe A et al. Combined surgical excision and radiation therapy for keloid treatment. J Craniofac Surg 2007; 18: 1164–9.
61. Alster TS. Laser treatment of hypertrophic scars, keloids, and striae. Dermatol Clin 1997; 15: 419–29.
62. Bouzari N, Davis SC, Nouri K. Laser treatment of keloids and hypertrophic scars. Int J Dermatol 2007; 46: 80–8.
63. Smit JM, Bauland CG, Wijnberg DS, Spawen PHM. Pulsed dye laser treatment, a review of indications and outcome based on published trials. Br J Plast Surg 2005; 58: 981–7.
64. Dierickx C, Goldman MP, Fitzpatrick RE. Laser treatment of erythematous/hypertrophic and pigmented scars in 26 patients. Plast Reconstr Surg 1995; 95: 84–90.
65. Alster TS, Kurban AK, Grove GL, Grove MJ, Tan OT. Alteration of argon laser-induced scars by the pulsed dye laser. Lasers Surg Med 1993; 13: 68–373.
66. Lipper GM, Perez M. Nonablative acne scar reduction after a series of treatments with a short-pulsed 1,064-nm neodymium:YAG laser. Dermatol Surg 2006; 32: 998–1006.
67. Berman B, Flores F. The treatment of hypertrophic scars and keloids. Eur J Dermatol 1998; 8: 591–5.
68. Nedelec B, Shankowsky H, Scott PG et al. Myofibroblasts and apoptosis in human hypertrophic scars: the effect of interferon-alpha2b. Surgery 2001; 130: 798–808.
69. Wang J, Jiao H, Stewart TL et al. Improvement in postburn hypertrophic scar after treatment with IFN-alpha2b is associated with decreased fibrocytes. J Interferon Cytokine Res 2007; 27: 921–30.
70. Hosnuter M, Payasli C, Isikdemir A, Tekerekoglu B. The effects of onion extract on hypertrophic and keloid scars. J Wound Care 2007; 16: 251–4.
71. Ho WS, Ying SY, Chan PC, Chan HH. Use of onion extract, heparin, allantoin gel in prevention of scarring in Chinese patients having laser removal of tattoos: a prospective randomized controlled trial. Dermatol Surg 2006; 32: 891–6.
72. Surh YJ, Na HK. Cyclooxygenase-2 as a putative target for cancer chemoprevention by some anti-inflammatory phytochemicals., in Essential Fatty Acids and Eicosanoids., Huang YS, Lin SJ, Huang PC, ed. AOCS Press: Champaign, Illinois, 2002: 146.
73. Phan TT, See P, Tran E et al. Suppression of insulin-like growth factor signalling pathway and collagen expression in keloid-derived fibroblasts by quercetin: its therapeutic potential use in the treatment and/or prevention of keloids. Br J Dermatol 2003; 148: 544–52.
74. Seo T, Blaner WS, Deckelbaum RJ. Omega-3 fatty acids: Molecular approaches to optimal biological outcomes. Curr Opin Lipidol 2005; 16: 11–8.
75. Larsson SC, Kumlin M, Ingelman-Sundberg M, Wolk A. Dietary long-chain n-3 fatty acids for the prevention of cancer: A review of potential mechanisms. Am J Clin Nutr 2004; 79: 935–45.

4 Topical therapy for acne scarring
James Q Del Rosso and Grace K Kim

CLINICAL SIGNIFICANCE OF ACNE VULGARIS AND ACNE SCARRING

Acne vulgaris (acne) is the most common skin disorder encountered by dermatologists in ambulatory practice, accounting for 11.3% of visits to non-Federal office—based on dermatologists practicing in the United States in 2005.(1) In one comprehensive study of individuals living in the United States aged 1 to 74 years, the prevalence of acne was determined to be 68 per 1,000 for both sexes, 70.4 per 1,000 for men, and 65.8 per 1,000 for women.(2) Other reports have suggested that acne affects 34% to 90% of males and 27% to 80% of females at some point during their lifetime, with the peak incidence reported to be between the ages of 14 and 17 years for females and 16 and 19 years for males.(3, 4) Although adolescents represent the population that is predominantly affected by acne, postteenage acne is not uncommon. One study evaluating patients with a mean age of 39.5 years (age range 25–58 years) reported the presence of active acne in 3% of males and 12% of females.(5) With regard to acne type and/or severity, the prevalence of cystic acne was determined in one analysis to be 1.9 per 1,000 for both sexes, 3.3 per 1,000 for males, and 0.6 per 1,000 for females.(2)

Although prevalence rates for acne vary among different epidemiologic reports depending on the methodology used for analysis, the bottom line is that acne is a very common disorder. Available publications likely underestimate the true prevalence rates of acne and its associated sequelae. This is because the epidemiologic data are based predominantly on those patients who attend dermatology clinics for acne treatment, with only up to 16% of individuals with visible facial acne estimated to actually seek therapy from a physician.(4, 6)

Due to the widespread prevalence of acne, both psychosocial and physical sequelae of the disease are commonly encountered problems that affect many patients in an adverse manner.(4, 6) The negative psychosocial implications of acne are well documented and include association with both currently visible acne and sequelae such as scarring.(7, 8) Adverse psychosocial effects of acne that have been reported are social embarrassment, poor self-esteem, emotional debilitation, social isolation, avoidance of interpersonal interaction, diminished academic performance, altered perception of body image, anger, frustration, anxiety, depression, and suicidal ideation.(7–9) Persistent physical sequelae of acne that are distressing to many patients include postinflammatory hyperpigmentation (PIH), postinflammatory erythema (PIE), and various types of scarring. Acne scarring represents the form of permanent sequelae from acne that is overall the most challenging to treat as outcomes may be variable, and the extent of improvement is usually only partial, depending on the type and extent of scarring that is present.(4, 6, 10, 11)

It is not surprising that acne is a common reason for a dermatologic office visit and that the disease produces negative psychosocial impact for many patients, as 97% of acne cases involve the face.(12) Truncal acne affects approximately half of all cases of acne presenting to a dermatology practice, with only 3% of acne cases involving only the trunk.(12) Over 70% of patients with truncal acne desire treatment for the trunk.(12) Therefore, although emphasis is placed on facial acne in terms of clinical and epidemiologic studies, both active acne and sequelae such as scarring that affects the trunk may also cause significant psychological distress for patients. Postacne scarring is significant in that its presence is particularly devastating to some patients and may in certain cases be a risk factor for suicidal ideation.(13)

PREVALENCE OF ACNE SCARRING

Epidemiologic data on acne scarring is limited, and the true prevalence is believed to be unknown.(14) One study reported acne scarring in 14% of women and 11% of men among 749 patients aged between 25 and 58 years.(5) Other publications suggest that between 30% and 95% of patients with acne develop some form of associated scarring.(6, 15) Additionally, a variety of clinical presentations of acne scarring may occur, with some patients demonstrating more than one type of scarring.(4, 6, 10, 11) Although atrophic scarring appears to be the most common type associated with acne, good epidemiologic data are not available on the relative prevalence rates of different types of acne scarring.(4, 16, 17)

IMPORTANCE OF EARLY TREATMENT FOR ACNE TO REDUCE THE RISK OF ACNE SCARRING

Scarring may occur early regardless of the severity of acne.(6) Although acne scarring is likely to be associated more often with nodulocytic acne and a greater intensity of visible inflammation, acne scarring may occur in cases with only superficial forms of acne, especially when effective treatment for acne is delayed.(6, 17)

Treatment delay is a significant problem in the management of acne and the prevention of physical sequelae such as scarring and dyschromias.(4) With the advent of multiple over-the-counter treatments that have limited efficacy, options promoted on television or on the internet that are poorly substantiated, and nonconventional therapies through sources not supervised by a knowledgeable physician, patients often use therapies for acne that are either ineffective, are not properly correlated with the severity of their disease, and are not optimally monitored. As a result, their acne persists or worsens, allowing for additional development of new acne lesions, thus prolonging their psychological distress and increasing the risk

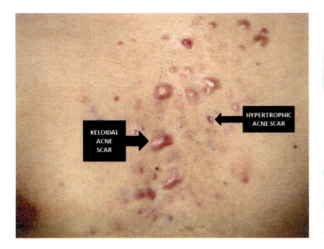

Figure 4.1 Hypertrophic Acne Scars and Keloidal Acne Scars.

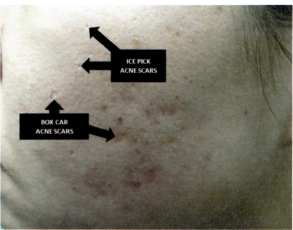

Figure 4.2 Ice Pick Acne Scars and Boxcar Acne Scars.

of scarring. One study showed that overall, approximately 16% of patients with acne seek proper treatment, and among those seeking such help, 74% wait greater than 12 months, 12% wait 6 to 12 months, 6% wait 6 months, and only 7% wait less than 3 months to be seen professionally for therapy of their acne.(18)

EVOLUTION OF ACNE SCARRING
Acne scarring occurs subsequent to visible resolution of deep inflammation. However, scarring may develop even when visible inflammation is minimal and at sites previously affected only by superficial inflammatory acne lesions.(6, 17) Proliferation of *Propionibacterium acnes* plays a pivotal role in the stimulation of innate immune response and the development of inflammation in acne.(19–21) Inflammation in acne is often initiated before rupture of the follicular wall; however, loss of wall integrity further amplifies the intensity of perifollicular inflammation.(19, 22) In addition, with dermal exposure of *P acnes*, activation of both the classic and alternative complement pathways occur.(19, 22) Incomplete containment of perifollicular inflammation secondary to follicular rupture may lead to formation of multichanneled fistulous tracts, open comedones, and/or ice-pick scars.(19, 22)

The ultimate appearance of acne scars relates to the extent and the depth of the inflammation.(4, 16, 17) When the preceding inflammation extends significantly into the dermis, degradation of the supporting matrix may be extensive, leading to a greater potential for scarring. Fibrosis and varying degrees of change in skin texture ensue after collagen and other dermal matrix components are damaged by the inflammation of acne. Over the next several months, deposition of new matrix and collagen synthesis occurs during the remodeling phase. Epidermal damage does not result in scarring but may produce persistent erythema or dyschromia, the latter most evident as foci of brown hyperpigmentation in individuals with darker skin types.

Ultimately, the amount, type, and depth of scarring are dependent on the location, nature, and intensity of the response to inflammation of the individual host.(17) However, it is not clear why some acne scars are atrophic in nature and others are hypertrophic, or why some individuals are more likely to form specific types of acne scars and not other types.(14, 16, 17) Acne scars have been generally classified into those involving *tissue loss* (atrophic) and those that produce *tissue excess* (hypertrophic).(10, 14, 16) Hypertrophic acne scars may be either *hypertrophic* or *keloidal* in nature.(10, 16) By definition, hypertrophic acne scars remain reasonably within the confines of the preexisting acne lesion, whereas keloidal acne scars extend markedly beyond the original site of the preexisting acne lesion (Figure 4.1).(10, 16, 17)

The major clinical types of atrophic scars are ice-pick scars (Figure 4.2), rolling or superficial and deep soft scars (Figure 4.3), and boxcar or depressed fibrotic scars (Figures 4.2 and 4.4) (Table 4.1).(4, 11, 14, 16) Why certain types of atrophic scars develop as opposed to others in a given patient is not known. However, familial tendency, genetic traits, both autosomal dominant and recessive, and anatomic factors influence the tendency to form keloidal-type scars.(4) Propensity for scarring has been correlated with a personal history of positivity for HLA B14, HLA BW16, HLA BW35, and HLA BW21.(23) Anatomically, hypertrophic acne scars, especially the keloidal-type, occur most commonly on the chest, back, and shoulders.(4) Potential pathophysiologic associations with the development of hypertrophic acne scars include altered expression of transforming growth factor-beta-1 (TGF-beta$_1$), platelet-derived growth factor, matrix metalloproteinases (MMPs), interleukin-1-alpha, carboxypeptidase A, prostaglandin D2, tryptase, and histamine, as well as altered microvascular regeneration.(4, 24, 25) TGF-beta$_1$ and TGF-beta$_2$ have been shown to be highly expressed in keloid-derived fibroblasts as compared with normal control fibroblasts,

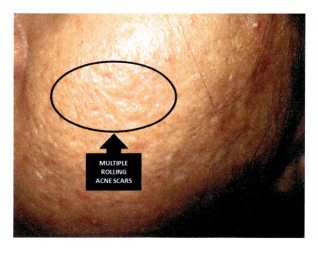

Figure 4.3 Multiple Rolling Acne Scars.

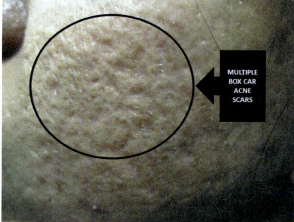

Figure 4.4 Multiple Boxcar Acne Scars.

Table 4.1 Classification of Acne Scars.

Scar Type	Clinical Features	Comments
Atrophic		
Ice pick	Narrow (<2 mm), deep, sharply marginated epithelial tracts, and conical or cyclindrical shape	Extend vertically into deep dermis or subcutis; depth reaches below level achieved by conventional resurfacing options
Rolling (superficial and deep soft scars)	Usually wider than 4–5 mm, shallow, anchored to subcutis by fibrosis (subdermal tethering)	Subdermal tethering causes superficial shadowing effect; subdermal anchoring fibrosis precludes treatment from above surface
Boxcar (depressed fibrotic scars)	Flat, u-shaped base; sharply marginated vertical edges; broader than ice-pick scars; round, polygonal, or linear shape; shallow (0.1–0.5 mm) or deep (>0.5 mm)	Usually broad; vary in size, shape, and depth; shallow types within depth reached by resurfacing treatments
Follicular macular atrophy	Perifollicular, soft, white macules; may be numerous; usually 2–4 mm in size	Perifollicular elastolysis; most common on trunk and/or upper arms and shoulders
Hypertrophic		
Hypertrophic	Raised, excess proliferation of fibrotic tissue, remain reasonably within confines of the preexisting acne lesion	Usually asymptomatic; most commonly seen on chest, back, and/or shoulders
Keloidal	Raised, excess proliferation of fibrotic tissue, extends obviously beyond the focus of the preexisting acne lesion	May be symptomatic (pruritus, pain); most commonly seen on chest, back, and/or shoulders

and the injection of TGF-beta$_1$ into athymic mice has produced the formation of keloid-like nodules.(17, 18) How these different potential pathophysiologic mechanisms correlate with the development of acne scarring is not entirely known; however, further research in this area may lead to the development of better therapies to treat or prevent hypertrophic acne scarring.

A distinctive form of acne scarring, *follicular macular atrophy*, is almost always seen on the trunk and/or upper arms.(14) This form of acne scarring presents as small, white, perifollicular, soft macules, which may sometimes be very numerous.

Follicular macular atrophy is believed to be the same entity as perifollicular elastolysis, as histologically there is marked loss of elastic tissue around affected follicles.(14)

It is important to recognize that PIE, a common residual finding after resolution of inflammatory acne lesions in fair-skinned individuals, may take months to fade after palpable inflammatory acne lesions dissipate (Figure 4.5).(17) PIE is often confused with acne scars by patients; however, the eventual development of visible scarring at sites of prior PIE is variable, necessitating final evaluation after the erythema fades.

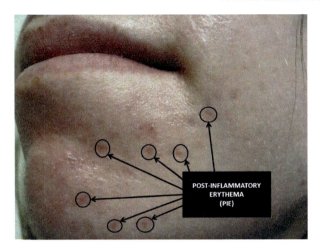

Figure 4.5 Postinflammatory Erythema (PIE).

INFLAMMATORY MECHANISMS, ACNE, AND ACNE SCARRING

More recent information on molecular mechanisms associated with inflammation in acne shed light on how specific therapies may be helpful in reducing acne lesions and potentially preventing acne scarring. The transcription factors, nuclear factor-kB (NK-kB), and activator protein-1 (AP-1) are activated in acne lesions, leading to upregulation of target gene products, inflammatory cytokines and matrix-degrading MMPs that serve as molecular mediators of inflammation and collagen degradation in acne lesions *in vivo*.(26) AP-1 has been shown to be activated in severe acne lesions.(26) After initiation of AP-1 activation, transcription of AP-1-regulated genes are increased. This leads to augmented production of several MMPs, such as MMP-1 (interstitial collagenase, collagenase-1), MMP-8 (neutrophil collagenase, collagenase 2), MMP-9 (92 kd gelatinase, collagenase 4), and MMP-13 (collagenase 3).(27) Each of these MMPs are involved with a variety of functions, including degradation of mature collagen and initiation of site-specific cleavage of type I and other fibrillar collagens (MMP-1), initiation of collagen degradation (MMP-8, MMP-13), and degradation of native fibrillar type-I and type-III collagen (MMP-1, MMP-8, MMP-13).(27) In addition, MMP-8 may be secreted by neutrophils that permeate the perifollicular region leading to dermal matrix degradation.(26, 27) *In vivo* analysis has shown that MMP-1, MMP-3, and MMP-9 are elevated in inflammatory acne lesions as compared to noninvolved facial controls.(26)

The degradation of dermal matrix is followed by a sequence of synthesis and repair of new collagen and other components of the surrounding dermal support network, which may sometimes be random and imperfect.(15) Visible acne scarring may occur if the cycles of upregulation of MMPs that degrade collagen and dermal matrix, and subsequent procollagen synthesis, are prolonged.(26) In the alternative, the resultant organization and composition of new collagen formation and extracellular matrix often produces dermal microdefects that are clinically undetectable; therefore, no visible scarring occurs.(26) The ability of certain agents used to treat acne to modulate different components of the inflammatory cascade explains the potential of these agents to prevent acne scarring if they are appropriately utilized for acne treatment.(28)

TOPICAL AGENTS USED FOR TREATMENT OF ACNE SCARRING

The vast majority of information on the treatment of acne scarring relates to the use of physical modalities and surgical procedures, such as dermabrasion, chemical peeling, tissue augmentation, laser resurfacing, nonablative laser techniques, radiofrequency, punch excision, punch elevation, elliptical excision, subscision, and debulking.(3, 4, 10, 11, 16, 17, 29) Unfortunately, there is a conspicuous absence of data on topical agents shown to be effective for the treatment of acne scars that are already present.(4, 10, 11, 16, 17, 30) Several topical agents have been sporadically mentioned, including vitamin A, E, C, zinc, and others, although none have been substantiated by scientifically acceptable clinical trials and none are generally accepted in current acne treatment guidelines as recommended therapies.(4, 31)

When discussing the use of topical agents for treatment of acne scars, it is very important to differentiate therapeutic benefit in reducing the development of acne scarring versus treatment of acne scars that are already present. Although long-term studies are lacking, clinical observation suggests that early and consistent treatment of acne that is appropriately correlated with the severity of disease, and properly adjusted if severity worsens, is successful in preventing the development of acne scars.(28) The therapeutic approach in a given patient utilizes topical agents (i.e., benzoyl peroxide, antibiotic, retinoid), often in combination, along with systemic therapy (i.e., oral antibiotic, hormonal agent), if warranted, based on acne severity.(31) The major objective of treatment at the time the patient presents initially with an acne flare is to select a treatment regimen that will result in adequate control of acne, with marked reduction or resolution of both inflammation and comedo development.(31, 32) Continuation of acne treatment once the disease process has improved is a vital component of successful management.(31) Long-term maintenance therapy controls both visible and subclinical inflammation and would be expected to reduce both acne lesions and acne scarring over time. As inflammation starts very early in the course of acne lesion development, active maintenance therapy for acne serves an important preventative therapeutic role, and a reduced potential for acne scarring would be an expected benefit of such therapy.(33)

TOPICAL RETINOIDS AND ACNE SCARRING

Among the topical agents used to treat acne vulgaris, topical retinoids, including tretinoin, adapalene, and tazarotene, exhibit several modes of antiinflammatory activity that theoretically

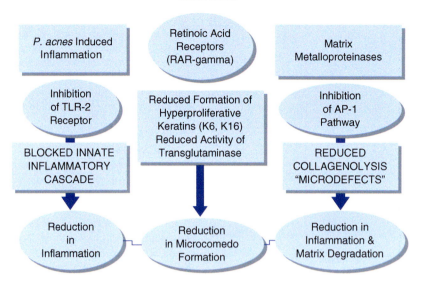

Figure 4.6 Topical Retinoids—Mechanisms of Action and Impact on Pathophysiology.

would appear to reduce the potential for development of acne scarring (Figure 4.6). These topical retinoids diminish the innate immune response stimulated by *P acnes* through downregulation of toll-like receptor-2 (TLR-2) located on perifollicular monocytes.(34, 35) Topical retinoids have also been shown to exhibit antiinflammatory and antiproliferative activities through inhibition of AP-1 activation.(36–38) Based on these reported mechanisms of action, topical retinoids blunt the inflammatory cascade early in its course by diminishing the innate immune response to *P acnes* and reduce the potential for dermal matrix degradation by inhibiting AP-1 activation, both of which should result in a diminished potential for acne scarring. Although data on prevention of acne scarring specifically is lacking, clinical studies on maintenance therapy with a topical retinoid alone for 12 to 16 weeks, and long-term monotherapy for up to 52 weeks, demonstrate that continued application of a topical retinoid results in the continual progressive reduction in both inflammatory and noninflammatory acne lesions.(39–41) As acne lesion reduction continues, it would be expected that acne scarring would also be reduced.

Whether or not the use of topical retinoids improves acne scars that are already present has not been evaluated or quantified in an appropriately controlled study.(42) Yet topical retinoids, such as tretinoin, have been shown to decrease the synthesis of MMPs and increase dermal procollagen and collagen synthesis, and hence may provide some benefit in preventing scar development and potentially reduce the extent of scar formation that is in progress ("unfixed scarring").(43–46) Topical retinoid therapy may possibly produce some smoothing of skin around areas of acne scarring through treatment of underlying acne and reduction in inflammation.(42) However, there is no cogent evidence demonstrating that topical retinoids reduce scars that are already fully formed in the dermis ("fixed scarring"). In addition, the effect of topical retinoids on different clinical presentations of acne scars, including both the atrophic and hypertrophic types, has not been evaluated.

TOPICAL ANTIMICROBIAL AGENTS AND ACNE SCARRING
There is no data that directly evaluate the impact of topical antimicrobial agents, such as benzoyl peroxide (BP), and antibiotics on acne scarring. These agents do, however, exhibit antiinflammatory activity through reduction in *P acnes*, and BP also exhibits moderate comedolytic activity.(28, 47) In addition, macrolide antibiotics, such as erythromycin, have been shown to inhibit neutrophil chemotaxis, suggesting that a direct antiinflammatory effect may also be operative.(48) It is generally anticipated that as long as inflammation and acne lesions are significantly reduced by application of topical antimicrobial therapy the potential for development of acne scarring would be diminished.

TOPICAL CORTICOSTEROIDS AND ACNE SCARRING
Intralesional triamcinolone injection for treatment of hypertrophic and keloidal scars is well established based on clinical experience, including for acne scarring.(4) Repeated injections may be needed depending on the size, thickness, and location of the scar. Use of topical corticosteroid therapy, either with or without occlusion, produces variable and inconsistent results in terms of reduction in hypertrophic or keloidal scarring, but may be helpful for short-term relief of associated pruritus, when present. It is likely to be more effective if a high-potency topical corticosteroid is used as compared to a low-potency formulation. Long-term topical corticosteroid application is not recommended as local side effects, such as atrophy and telangiectasia,

may occur in the skin surrounding the area of the scar due to contiguous application or spread of the topical agent.

TOPICAL COSMECEUTICALS AND ACNE SCARRING
The breaking open of capsules containing vitamin E and massaging the contents into scars is a common practice among the lay public. There is no scientific evidence that this practice is effective in either reducing scars that are already present or in preventing scar formation.(42)

Concern has been raised regarding whether or not application of growth factors such as TGF-beta could contribute to development of hypertrophic or keloidal scars.(49) At present, there is no clinical evidence that cutaneous application of growth factors, such as TGF-beta, induce abnormal scar development.(49) Anecdotal observations have not detected an association with the production of hypertrophic scars, keloidal scars, or abnormal wound-healing response despite widespread use of topical products containing TGF-beta.(49)

CONCLUSION
Scar formation as a sequelae of acne is a dynamic process. This process begins with inflammation within the pilosebaceous unit, which starts subclinically, and usually progresses to a visible inflammatory lesion that may be deep or superficial in nature. The next step is dermal matrix degradation that occurs as a response to inflammation. The net result is finally dependent on what transpires during the dermal remodeling phase, as new collagen and other supporting matrix components are produced, and subsequently, as these components are incorporated into the dermal network during the organization phase. After this process is finished, the repair process is relatively complete, and any resulting fibrosis (and possibly visible scar formation) that has occurred is then fixed. Therefore, whether or not a given topical agent is helpful for prevention or treatment of acne scars is dependent on whether or not the agent is capable of reducing the extent of scar development by appropriately modulating one or more steps in the acne-repair process.

REFERENCES
1. Weinstock M, Boyle M. Statistics of interest to the dermatologist. In: Year Book of Dermatology and Dermatologic Surgery. Thiers BH, Lang PG, eds. Philadephia: Elsevier-Mosby, 2008: 41.
2. Johnson M, Roberts J. Skin conditions and related need for medical care among persons 1–74 years, United States, 1971–1974. Washington, DC: US Department of Health, Education and Welfare, Vital and Health Statistics, Series 11, No. 212, November 2008.
3. Fien S, Ballard C, Nouri K. Multiple modalities to treat acne: a review of lights, lasers and radiofrequency. Cosmet Dermatol 2004; 17: 789–93.
4. Rivera A. Acne scarring: a review and current treatment modalities. J Am Acad Dermatol 2008; 59: 659–76.
5. Goulden V, Stables G, Cunliffe W. Prevalence of facial acne in adults. J Am Acad Dermatol 1999; 41: 577–80.
6. Goodman G. Management of post-acne scarring: what are the options for treatment? Am J Clin Dermatol 2000; 1: 3–17.
7. Ginsburg I. The psychosocial impact of skin disease: an overview. Dermatol Clin 1996; 14: 473–84.
8. Koo J. The psychosocial impact of acne: patients' perceptions. J Am Acad Dermatol 1995; 32(Suppl): S26–S30.
9. Schacter R, Pantel E, Glassman G. Acne vulgaris and psychological impact on high school students. NY State J Med 1971; 24: 2886–99.
10. Jemec G, Jemec B. Acne: treatment of scars. Clinics in Dermatol 2004; 22: 434–8.
11. Frith M, Harmon C. Acne scarring: current treatment options. Dermatol Nursing 2006; 18: 139–42.
12. Del Rosso J, Bikowski J, Baum E, Hawkes S. A closer look at truncal acne vulgaris: prevalence, severity, and clinical significance. J Drugs Dermatol 2007; 6: 597–600.
13. Cotteril J, Cunliffe W. Suicide in dermatological patients. Br J Dermatol 1997; 137: 246–50.
14. Cunliffe W. Clinical features of acne. In: Acne, 1st edn. Cunliffe WC, ed. Chicago: Martin Dunitz-Year Book, 1989: 20–32.
15. Cunliffe WJ. The sebaceous gland and acne-40 years on. Dermatology 1996; 196: 9–15.
16. Jacob C, Dover J, Kaminer M. Acne scarring: a classification system and review of treatment options. J Am Acad Dermatol 2001; 45: 109–17.
17. Kim G, Del Rosso J. Acne scarring: treatment and management. Cosmet Dermatol 2009 (accepted for publication).
18. Tan J, Vasey T, Fung K. Beliefs and perceptions of patients with acne. J Am Acad Dermatol 2001; 44: 439–45.
19. Farrar M, Ingham E. Acne: inflammation. Clinics in Dermatol 2004; 22: 380–4.
20. Vowels B, Yang S, Leyden J. Induction of proinflammatory cytokines by a soluble factor of Propionibacterium acnes: implications for chronic inflammatory acne. Infect Imunnol 1995; 63: 3158–65.
21. Kim J, Ochoa M, Krutzik S. Activation of toll-like receptor-2 in acne triggers inflammatory cytokine responses. J Immunol 2002; 169: 1535–41.
22. Webster G, Leyden J, Nilsson U. Complement activation in acne vulgaris: consumption of complement by comedones. Infect Immun 1979; 26: 183–6.
23. Oluwasanmi J, Otusanya M. Human leucocyte antigens (HLA) and keloids. W Afr J Med 1983; 2: 127–30.
24. Smith P, Mosiello G, Deluca L. TGF-beta2 activates proliferative scar fibroblasts. J Surg Res 1999; 82: 319–23.
25. Campaner AB, Ferreira LM, Gragnani A. Upregulation of TGF-beta-1 expression may be necessary but is not sufficient for excessive scarring. J Invest Dermatol 2006; 126: 1168–76.
26. Kang S, Cho S, Chung J et al. Inflammation and extracellular matrix degradation mediated by activated transcription

factora nuclear factor-kB and activator protein-1 in inflammatory acne lesions in vivo. Am J of Path 2005; 166: 1691–9.

27. Birkedal-Hansen H, Moore W, Bodden M. Matrix metalloproteinases: a review. Crit Rev Oral Biol Med 1993; 4: 197–250.

28. Layton A. Optimal management of acne to prevent scarring and psychological sequelae. Am J Clin Dermatol 2001; 2: 135–41.

29. Orentreich N, Durr N. Rehabilitation of acne scarring. Dermatol Clin 1983; 1: 405–13.

30. Cunliffe W. Treatment of acne scars. In: Acne, 1st edn. Cunliffe WC, ed. Chicago: Martin Dunitz-Year Book, 1989: 337–53.

31. Gollnick H, Cunliffe W, Berson D et al. Global alliance to improve outcomes in acne. J Am Acad Dermatol 2003; 49 (Suppl 1): S1–S37.

32. Del Rosso J, Kim G. Optimizing use of oral antibiotics in acne vulgaris. Dermatol Clin 2009; 27: 33–42.

33. Jeremy A, Holland D, Roberts S. Inflammatory events are involved in acne lesion initiation. J Invest Dermatol 2003; 121: 20–7.

34. Liu P, Krutzik S, Kim J. Cutting edge. All-trans retinoic acid down-regulates TLR2 expression and function. J Immunol 2005; 174: 2467–70.

35. Tenaud I, Khammari A, Dreno B. In vitro modulation of TLR-2, CD1d and IL-10 by adapalene on normal skin and acne inflammatory lesions. Exp Dermatol 2007; 16: 500–6.

36. Sorg O, Antille C, Saurat J. Retinoids, other topical vitamins, and antioxidants. In: Photoaging. Rigel DS, Weiss RA, Lim HW, Dover JS, eds. New York: Marcel Dekker, 2004: 97–101.

37. Benkoussa M, Brand C, Delmotte M. Retinoic acid receptors inhibit AP-1 activation by regulating extracellular signal-related kinase and CBP recruitment to an AP-1 responsive promoter. Mol Cel Biol 2002; 22: 4522–34.

38. Nagpal S, Chandraratna R. Recent developments in receptor-selective retinoids. Curr Pharm Des 2000; 6: 919–31.

39. Thiboutot D, Shalita A, Yamauchi P et al. Adapalene gel. 0.1%, as maintenance therapy for acne vulgaris: a randomized, controlled, investigator-blinded follow-up of a recent combination study. Arch Dermatol 2006; 142: 597–602.

40. Leyden J, Thiboutot D, Shalita A et al. Comparison of tazarotene and minocycline maintenance therapies in acne vulgaris: a multicenter, double-blind, randomized, parallel-group study. Arch Dermatol 2006; 142: 605–12.

41. Weiss J, Thiboutot D, Hwa J, Liu Y, Graeber M. Long-term safety and efficacy of adapalene 0.3% gel. J Drugs Dermatol 2008; 7(Suppl 6): S24–S28.

42. Draelos Z. Acne cosmeceutical myths. In: Cosmeceuticals, 2nd edn. Draelos ZD, ed. Philadelphia: Saunders-Elsevier, 2009: 180–1.

43. Chen S, Kiss I, Tramposch K. Effects of all-trans retinoic acid on UVB-irradiated and non-irradiated hairless mouse skin. J Invest Dermatol 1992; 98: 248–54.

44. Griffiths C, Russman A, Mjmudar G. Restoration of collagen formation in photodamaged human skin by tretinoin (retinoic acid). N Engl J Med 1993; 329: 530–5.

45. Fisher G, Wang Z, Datta S. Pathophysiology of premature skin aging induced by ultraviolet light. N Engl J Med 1997; 337; 1419–28.

46. Kang S, Bergfeld W, Gottlieb A et al. Long-term efficacy and safety of tretinoin emollient cream 0.05% in the treatment of photodamaged facial skin: a two-year, randomized, placebo-controlled trial. Am J Clin Dermatol 2005; 6: 245–53.

47. Tanghetti E, Popp K. A current review of topical benzoyl peroxide: new perspectives on formulation and utilization. Dermatol Clin 2009; 27: 17–24.

48. Sugihara E. Effect of macrolide antibiotics on neutrophil function in human peripheral blood. Kansenshogaku Zasshi 1997; 71: 329–36.

49. Draelos Z. Endogenous growth factors as cosmeceuticals. In: Cosmeceuticals, 2nd edn. Draelos ZD, ed. Philadelphia: Saunders-Elsevier, 2009: 141–2.

5 Superficial peeling
Maria Pia De Padova and Antonella Tosti

KEY FEATURE BOX

- Very useful for treating pigmented macular scars
- Useful for improving boxcar scars
- Improve active acne lesions
- Can be utilized for dark skin

INTRODUCTION

Superficial peelings include salicylic acid, 25% to 30%; glycolic acid, 70%; piruvic acid, 40% and/or 50% to 60%; trichloracetic acid, 20% to 30%; and combination of salicylic acid or Jessner peel with trichloracetic acid.

Supercial peelings are utilized to induce a damage limited to the epidermis and papillary dermis. This results in epidermal regeneration and postinflammatory collagen neoformation. Because their potency is mild, repeated treatment are required to obtain the desired effects. Their efficacy is limited to macular and mild atrophic scars (boxcar scars).

Choice of peel depends on skin type and type of scars.(1, 2, 3) The most utilized agent for treatment for mild acne scars is trichloracetic acid, alone or in combination with salicylic or glycolic acid. Piruvic acid or trichloracetic acid in combination with salicylic acid are good choices when acne scars are associated with active acne lesions. Piruvic acid is widely utilized for scars in Asian patients. Studies comparing efficacy of different superficial peels in acne scars are needed.

DIFFUSION OF THE TECHNIQUE

Superficial peels are widely utilized worldwide in both women and men. The relative safety of these peelings in dark phototypes explains their utilization in different races. Superficial peels can be utilized for acne scars in young as well middle-aged patients where they may also be helpful to improve photoaging.(4)

HISTORY

In 1882, Unna first described the keratolytic properties of salicylic acid, trichloracetic acid, and phenol. Treatment of acne scars, however, has been mostly approached with deep or medium-deep peelings.

The concept of utilizing repeated sessions of superficial peels instead of medium-deep peels in the treatment of scars is quite recent and most of the published literature describes the utilization of 70% glycolic acid.(5, 6, 7)

PATHOPHYSIOLOGY

The pathological changes of acne scars have common features with photoaging with flattening and thinning of epidermal rete ridges, dermal elastosis, and decreased collagen. Superficial peelings induce coagulation necrosis of the epidermis and papillary dermis. The inflammatory reaction has stimulatory effects on fibroblasts with new collagen production; this explains their efficacy on atrophic scars. The exfoliating effects and the increased epidermal turnover explain their efficacy on macular scars.(8)

TECHNOLOGY

Indications/Advantages/Disadvantages

Treatment of acne scars requires 4 to 7 sessions, with an interval of 30 to 40 days, with all peeling agents.

Choice of type of superficial peelings depends on type of scars, skin type, and skin thickness, which is influenced by previous topical treatments and environmental factors such as cold weather that increases peel penetration.

Salicylic acid 25–30 % followed by Trichloracetic acid 30%: patients with active acnes and boxcar scars/ most effective for patients with comedonic acnes and deeper scars. Provides a very homogeneous peel (Figure 5.1A,B).

Jessner's Solution followed by Trichloracetic acid 25%–30%: patients with active acnes and boxcar scars/ same indication as combination peeling with Salicylic acid and Trichloracetic acid.

Salicylic acid 25% followed by Trichloracetic acid 25%: patients with active acnes, superficial boxcar scars and macular scars/ less aggressive and then shorter postpeeling healing phase (Figure 5.2A,B, Figure 5.3).

Trichloracetic acid 25–30%: patients with boxcar scars without active lesions/25 and 30% concentrations can be used in the same patient to treat scars of different deep.

Salicylic acid 25%: patients with active acnes and macular scars/ very rapid effect/ safe in dark skin.

Glycolic acid 70%: macular scars especially in patients without active acne lesions/should be used with caution as may cause residual macular or atrophic scars due its fast and often not homogeneous penetration.

Piruvic acid 40–60% patients with active acnes, macular scars and very superficial boxcar scars. Very rapid effect on active acne lesions. Provides a very homogeneous peel. Improves skin texture.(9) (Figure 5.4A,B; Figure 5.5A,B)

Controindications

Controindications to superficial peelings include

- connective tissue disorders
- active skin disorders on the treatment sites
- history of treatment with systemic retinoids in the previous 4 months
- oral anticoagulant treatment
- pregnancy

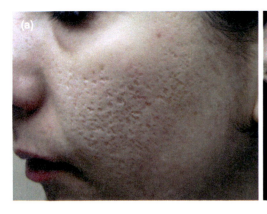
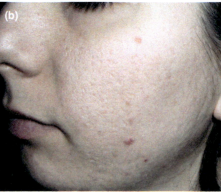

Figure 5.1 Boxcar scars before (A) and after (B) 5 sessions with combined 25% salycilic acid and 30% trichloracetic acid peeling. Note that scars are more superficial.

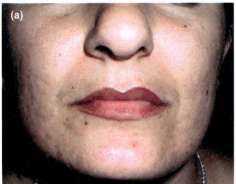
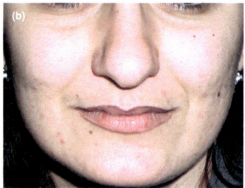

Figure 5.2 Boxcar scars before (A) and after (B) 5 sessions with 25% trichloracetic acid peeling.

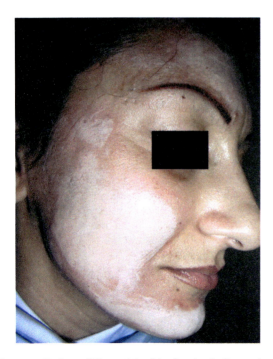

Figure 5.3 Patient of Figure 5.2, white frosting indicates that it is time to neutralize with cold water.

TECHNICAL PROCEDURE

Home preparation to peeling

This is essential to obtain uniform penetration and avoid postinflammatory hyperpigmentation. Prescribe topical products containing 1% to 2% salicylic acid or 2% to 3% pyruvic acid or 0.05% retinoic acid to be applied 3 times a week for 1 month. Prescribe 4% topical hydroquinone 3 times a week for 1 month. Application of these topicals should be interrupted 4 days before the procedure to avoid excessive penetration of the peeling agent.

Treatment with oral antivirals should be started 2 days before the procedure in patients with history of recurrent herpes simplex infections.

A detailed informed consent should be given to the patient at this time to give her/him the possibility of understanding the procedure and asking possible questions before treatment. We always provide written information about the procedure (Table 5.1). It is very important to explain clearly to the patient that superficial peels can improve but may not completely resolve acne scars to avoid excessive expectations.

Photographic documentation

It is mandatory to obtain good-quality pictures before starting the procedure. This is an essential documentation for follow-up and for possible medicolegal issues.(10)

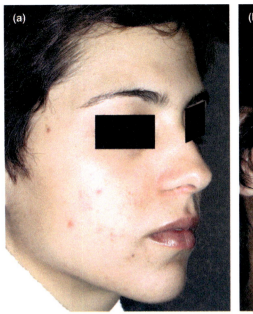
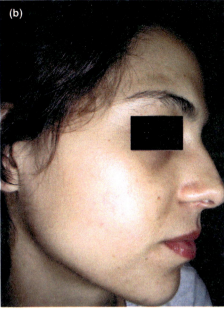

Figure 5.4 Macular scars before (A) and after (B) 4 sessions of 50% pyruvic acid peeling.

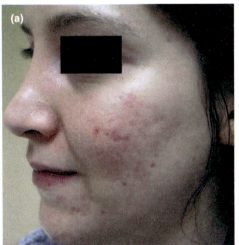
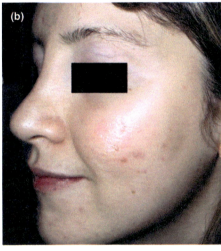

Figure 5.5 Active acne with macular scars before (A) and after (B) 4 sessions of pyruvic acid peeling.

Table 5.1 Patient's information about chemical peeling.

- Superficial peels are a cosmetic procedure that has the purpose of exfoliating the skin through the application of chemicals that induce skin irritation and damage.
- Expect severe burning during the procedure. This will usually last for 3 to 4 minutes.
- Expect skin redness for 2 to 3 days
- The skin will turn red brown and start to peel, 2 to 3 days after peeling. Though rare, you can expect blisters and crusts.
- The procedure can cause pigmented or white spots that are usually temporary and resolve in 1 to 3 months. In some skin types, however, these pigmentary changes may persist and require specific treatments.
- For the first week after procedure apply a moisturizer 3 to 4 times a day.
- Don't scratch or remove the scales as it may result in scarring.
- Avoid sun exposure, as it will cause development of pigmentary spots. Wear a high-protection sunscreen all the time for at least 2 months after procedure.
- Superficial peels improve the skin, but may not completely eliminate acnes scars
- You may need to repeat the procedure 3 to 6 times for optimal results.

Choice of agent/concentration

In patients with active acne lesions we suggest either a combination of salicylic acid and trichloracetic acid, a combination of Jessner's solution and trichloracetic acid or pyruvic acid.

For macular scars we suggest either pyruvic acid at 40% to 50%, salicylic acid at 25%, or glycolic acid at 70%.

Pyruvic acid is used at 40% 50% for macular scars, at 50% for superficial scars, and at 60% for boxcar scars.

Trichloracetic acid: If alone use the 30% concentration except for very superficial scars where it can be used at 25%. In combination peels, trichloracetic acid can be used at 25% to 30% as the first agent increases the penetration and, therefore, the peeling effect.

Concentrations depend also on the skin areas as periocular and perioral regions require lower concentrations or milder application of the peel.

Choice of formulation

All the chemicals utilized for superficial peelings are on the markets as solutions.

Some agents are also available in gels and pads.

In general, gel formulations have a slower penetration time and are easier to control. We personally prefer these formulations when available.

Peeling tray

The tray should include the peeling agents, the neutralizing solution (10% sodium carbonate), alcohol, acetone, cold water, gauzes, cotton-tipped applicators, disposable fan brushes, disposable hair caps, portable fun, zinc oxide cream, and total block sunscreen.

It is very important that the container of the peeling agent is clearly distinguishable from the container of the neutralizing solution and water to avoid possible confusion.

Skin cleaning

Before peeling, the skin should be cleaned to remove the hydrolipidic film and obtain optimal penetration. Alcohol or acetone can be utilized for this purpose.

Application

The patient should be seated in a comfortable position, wear a disposable hair cap, and be instructed to keep the eyes closed during the procedure.

A zinc oxide paste should be applied at the lip and eyelid commissures.

Always keep the container with the peeling agents on the side of the patient to avoid inadvertent dropping.

The modality of application depends on formulation. Liquids products are better applied using a fan brush; gel products can be applied with cotton-tipped applicators o gloved fingers.

Treatment should start from facial areas with thicker skin.

Apply the peeling agent on the forehead first, from side to side, 2 or 3 times and then do the same on the cheeks, the nose, and the chin. The periocular and perioral regions should be treated at last. For obtaining a homogeneous peeling, repeat the application in regions that do not show erythema or frosting.

Key factors for obtaining best results with superficial peelings in acne scars is to apply a strong pressure on the skin around the scar during treatment in order to enhance penetration of the peeling agent in the surrounding skin. This produces uplifting of the atrophic area.

For deep box scars, it is important to compress with the cotton tip the central region of the scar.(11)

Combined salicylic acid and trichloracetic acid peels: Apply the salicylic acid solution first. The solution should be left for 2 to 3 minutes until evaporation of the alcoholic vehicle. Using water or a moisturizing cream, remove the residual salicylic acid white power from the treated area. Apply the trichloracetic acid in solution or gel until frosting.

The optimal frost is white-pink for macular scars and white-gray for other scars. Use cold water to neutralize the peel and select degree of frosting.

Combined Jessner's solution / trichloracetic acid peels: Apply the Jessner's solution first and then follow the same modalities for the combined salycilic–tricholacetic acid peel.(12, 13)

Trichloracetic acid peel: Apply the trichloracetic acid in solution or gel until frosting (Figure 5.6). Use cold water to neutralize the peel and select degree of frosting (11, 14, 15).

Salicylic acid at 25%: The solution should be left for 2 to 3 minutes until evaporation of the alcoholic vehicle. Use a moisturizing cream to remove the residual salicylic acid white power from the treated area, as this improves penetration of salicylic acid in the skin. (16) (Figure 5.7)

Glycolic acid at 70%: The solution or gel should be left for 2 to 3 minutes until diffuse erythema develops and then neutralized with 10% sodium carbonate. Avoid development of frosting, as it may be source of postpeeling complications.(17, 18)

Pyruvic acid at 40% to 60%: The solution or gel should be left for 3 to 4 minutes or until frosting for boxcar scars. Use 10% sodium carbonate solution to neutralize the peeling.(19, 20, 21)

Immediate postpeel care

1. The patient will complain of burning a few seconds after beginning of the procedure.
2. The development of diffuse homogeneous erythema indicates epidermal penetration. (Figure 5.8)
3. Development of white frost indicates coagulative necrosis of the papillary dermis.(Figure 5.9A,B; Figure 5.10, Figure 5.11)
4. Development of gray-white frost indicates coagulative necrosis of the reticular dermis.(Figure 5.10)
5. The patient will develop diffuse erythema and edema about 1 hour after the end of the procedure.
6. Skin desquamation usually develops 3 to 4 days after peeling (Figure 5.11)

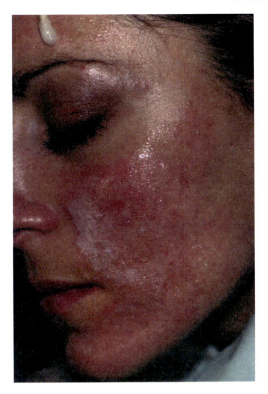

Figure 5.6 25% trichloracetic acid peeling in a gel formulation. Note homogeneous erythema and initial white frosting. Wait for homogeneous white frosting before neutralize.

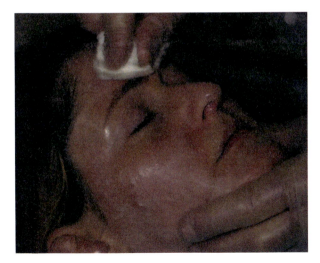

Figure 5.7 25% salycilic acid peeling. The white color is due to the residual salycilic acid power.

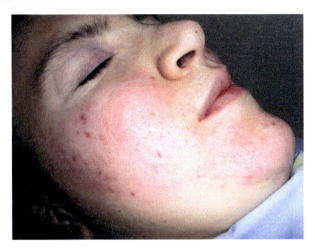

Figure 5.8 Patient of Figure 5.5 during procedure. The presence of homogeneous erythema indicates time of neutralization with 10% sodium carbonate solution.

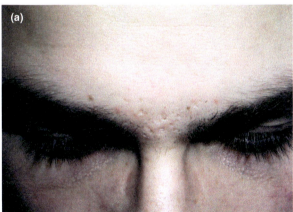

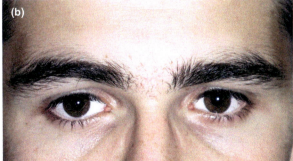

Figure 5.9 Boxcar scars and ice pick scars of the glabella before (A) and after (B) 4 sessions of 30% trichloracetic acid peeling.

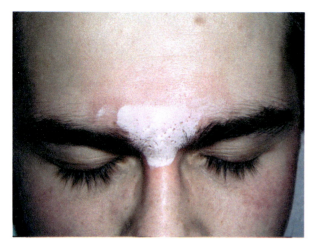

Figure 5.10 Patient of Figure 5.9, white frosting indicates that the agent has reached the reticular dermis.

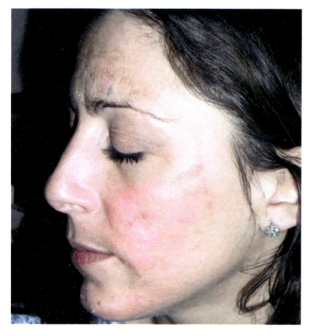

Figure 5.11 Patient of Figure 5.6, 3 days after the procedure. Note diffuse erythema and mild hyperpigmentation.

Postpeeling care

Apply a moisturizing cream containing a sun block and inform the patient to avoid sun exposure.

For the immediate postpeeling period the patient should apply a moisturizing cream 3 to 4 times a day and avoid to scratch or peel the skin. A mild skin cleanser can be utilized without rubbing.

In case of intense erythema prescribe a low-potency topical steroids for 2 to 3 days.

When riepithelization is complete, this usually takes 7 to 10 days, the patient can reassume application of topical products containing 1% to 2% salicylic acid, 2% to 3% pyruvic acid, or 0.05% retinoic acid and 4% topical hydroquinone to prepare the skin to the next procedure.

Patients with active acne lesions can use topical antibiotics and/or benzoyl peroxide.

The patient should regularly wear a total sun block between peeling sessions and up to 6 months after the last session.

Superficial peelings may temporarily worsen papulo-pustolar acne and some patients develop active papules and pustules in the immediate postpeeling period. These patients can be treated with systemic antibiotics as in the management of active acne.(22, 23)

MANAGEMENT OF SIDE EFFECTS AND COMPLICATIONS

Minor side effects

Minor side effects are common and include temporary swelling, burning, itching, dryness, skin hypersensitivity, transient hypo- or hyper-pigmentation.

All these side effects are transitory. Swelling, itching, and burning usually do not require treatment and resolve spontaneously in 1 week; a mild topical steroids can be given for 1 to 2 days in most severe cases.

Skin dryness and hypersensitivity may last for 2 weeks and just require frequent application of moisturizing creams.

Pigmentary changes may last between 3 and 4 weeks. In these patients, it is very important to completely avoid sun exposure. For hyperpigmented spots, bleaching agents such as 4% hydroquinone and 0.05% retinoic acid can be prescribed.

Complications and Management

Complications can be due to doctor or patient's responsibilities.

Doctor' s possible mistakes include choice of excessive concentrations or inadequate modality of application resulting in dishomogeneous penetration, accidental dropping of the peeling solution into the eyes, mouth, or other sensitive regions. The damage can be severe, especially with agents that require neutralization.

Permanent complications include corneal damage, atrophic or hypertrophyc scars, diffuse or spotted hypo or hyperpigmentation, patchy dishomogeneous areas of different skin color.

Atrophic scars can be treated with fillers. Hypertrophic scars can be treated with steroid injections and silicone dressing.

Prescribe bleaching agents for pigmentary changes. In patients with dishomogeneous skin color a few sessions of 40% pyruvic acid peeling or 5% retinoic acid peeling can be of help.

Herpes simplex reactivation may occur if prophylaxis has not been prescribed. In this case immediately start treatment with systemic antivirals.

Patients may not follow instructions as they frequently remove scales and crust to accelerate healing; this may result in prolonged erythema and possible dishomogeneous skin color. They may not avoid sun exposure and develop hyperpigmented areas.

OUTLOOK—FUTURE DEVELOPMENTS
Superficial peelings can be more widely utilized in combination with other treatments of acne scars such as needling, lasers, and fillers.

Evidence-based studies that evaluate efficacy of different superficial peelings in active acnes and scars are required.

SUMMARY FOR THE CLINICIAN BOX
Superficial peelings can be utilized both in active and inactive acne with scars.

Peelings treatment in active acne may prevent further scarring by reducing the inflammation.

Superficial peelings improve macular and superficial scars. They are not useful for ice-pick and rolling scars.

Choice of peeling should always take in account the following: type of skin, type of scars, and acne activity.

Skin preparation to peeling is essential for optimal homogeneity in penetration.

Application requires proper training for each peeling agent in order to avoid excessive penetration and possible complications.

Postpeeling care requires good cooperation from the patient, who needs to be well instructed on the purpose of treatment and expected effects of the peels, including minor side effects and possible complications (Table 5.1).

Some patients require repeated treatment sessions during the years as photoaging make atrophic scars more evident.

REFERENCES
1. Goodman GJ. Management of post-acne scarring: what are the options for treatment? Am J Clin Dermatol 2000; 1: 3–17.
2. Cunliffe WJ. Comedogenesis: some new aetiological, clinical and strategie. Br J Dermatol 2000; 142: 1084–91.
3. Jacob CI, Dover JS, Kaminer MS. Acne scarring: a classification system and review of treatment options. J Am Acad Dermatol 2001; 45: 109–17.
4. Makram M, Al Waiz. Medium-depth chemical peels in the treatment of acne scars in dark-skinned individuals. J Dermatol Surg 2002; 28: 383–7.
5. Ayres S. Superficial chemo-surgery in treating aging skin Arch Dermatol 1962; 85: 385–93.
6. Van Scott EJ, Yu RJ. Hyperkeratinization, corneocyte cohesion and alpha-hydroxy acids. J Am Acad Dermatol 1984; 11: 867–79.
7. Brody HJ, Hailey CW. Medium-depth chemical peeling of the skin: a variation of superficial chemosurgery. J Dermatol Surg Oncol 1986; 12: 1268–75.
8. James J, Stagnone MD. Superficial peeling. J Dermatol Surg Oncol 1989; 15: 924–30.
9. Griffin TD, Van Scott EJ, Maddin S. The use of pyruvic acid as a chemical peeling agent. J Dermatol Surg Oncol 1989; 15: 1316.
10. Goodman GJ, Baron JA. Post acne scarring -a qualitative global scarring grading system. Dermatol Surg 2006; 32: 1458–66.
11. Lee JB, Chung WG, Kwahck H, Lee KH. Focal treatment of acne scar whith trichloracetic acid: chemical reconstruction of skin scars method. Dermatol Surg 2002; 28(11): 1017–21.
12. Rubin MG. Manual of chemical peels: superficial and medium depth. J.B. Lippincott Company, Philadelphia, 1995: 79–88.
13. Moy LS, Peace S. Comparison of the effect of various chemical peeling agents in a mini pig model. Dermatol Surg 1996; 22: 429–32.
14. Harold J. Brody. Chemical Peeling and Resurfacing. 1997 2nd Ed. by Mosby.
15. Ghersetich I, Teofoli P, Gantcheva M, Ribuffo M, PudduP. Chemical peeling: how, when, why? J Eur Acad Dermatol venereal 1997; 8: 1.
16. Grimes PE. The safety and efficacy of salicylic acid chemical peels in darker racial-ethnic groups. Dermatol Surg 1999; 25(1): 18–22.
17. Wang CM, Huang CL, Hu CT, Chan HL. The effect of glycolic acid on the treatment of acne in Asian skin. Dermatol Surg 1997; 23: 23–9.
18. Erbagei Z, Akçali C. Biweekly serial glycolic acid peels vs. long-term daily use of topical low-strength glycolic acid in the treatment of atrophic acne scars. Int J Dermatol 2000; 39(10): 789–94.
19. Ghersetich I, De Padova MP. Peeling chimici, indicazioni e limiti. Dermatologia e Cosmesi. La Pelle, Anno VIII, Novembre (11) 2002: 43–5.
20. Cotellessa C, Manunta T, Ghersetich I et al. The use of pyruvic acid in the treatment of acne. J Eur Acad Dermatol Venereol 2004; 18(3): 275–8.
21. Berardesca E, Cameli N, Primavera G et al. Clinical and instrumental evaluation of skin improvement after treatment with a new 50% pyruvic Acid peel. Dermatol Surg 2006; 32(4): 526–31.
22. Tosti A, Grimes PE, De Padova MP. Altlas of chemical peels. Springer, 2006.
23. Furukawa F, Yamamoto Y. Recent advances in chemical peeling in Japan. J Dermatol 2006; 33: 655–61.

6 Medium depth and deep peeling
Marina Landau

KEY FEATURES

- Acne scars can not be effectively corrected by a single treatment modality. By combining modalities they can be significantly improved.
- Best results are achieved in older female patients, rather than in young males. Atrophic scars response better than ice-picked and hypertrophic ones.
- With deeper peels, more significant result are achieved.
- The degree of the frosting in TCA peel correlates with the depth of solution penetration.
- Full-face deep peels are carried out under full cardiopulmonary monitoring and intravenous hydration.

INTRODUCTION

Chemical peelings are a procedure used for cosmetic improvement of the skin or for treatment of some skin disorders. Although few years ago some have predicted the disappearance of chemical peels in favor of lasers, quite the opposite have occurred.(1) According to the official Web site of the American Society of Plastic Surgeons, there was 435% increase in chemical peels in 2005 versus 1992 with a total of 1 million procedures performed by the members (www.plasticsurgery.org).

Popularity of chemical peels is related to their versatility and relative simplicity. During the peeling procedure chemical exfoliating agent is applied to the skin to destruct portions of epidermis and/or dermis with subsequent regeneration and rejuvenation of the tissues. The peels are classified as superficial, medium, and deep according to the depth of penetration of the peeling solution. The depth of the peel determines patient's inconvenience during and after the procedure, healing time, the rate of the potential side effects, and the results.(2)

Acne is a common disease affecting almost 100% of youngsters.(3, 4) Acne settles in the vast majority by 20 to 25 years of age but 1% of males and 5% of females exhibit acne lesions at 40 years of age.(5) Scarring occurs early in the course of acne and may affect to some degree 95% of patients from both sexes.(6) Differences in the cell-mediated immune response are involved in the personal tendency to develop postacne scarring.(7)

Acne scars are debilitating and socially disabling for the individual. Treatment of acne scars presents a challenge for a physician. Usually they can not be effectively corrected by a single treatment modality because of their widely varied depth, width, and structure. By combining modalities significant improvement of the scarred skin is obtained.

HISTORY

As far back as 1905, surgical methods have been used to improve skin that has been scarred by facial acne. One hundred years ago two New York dermatologists, George MacKee and Florentine Karp, began using phenol peels for postacne scarring.(8) Thereafter, methods used to correct acne scars included dermatome dermaplaning (9, 10); dermabrasion(11–13); collagen implantation (14–16); demal overgrafting (17); punch excision, grafting, and elevation(18, 19); dermal grafting (20, 21); subcision (6, 22); laser resurfacing (23–29); microdermabrasion (30); dermasanding (31); and their combinations.(32–34)

But the mainstay of therapy for skin resurfacing continues to be chemical peels combined with skin abrasion.(35–39)

BASIC CHEMISTRY

Chemical peels in use to improve facial scarring include alpha hydroxyl acid peels, trichloroacetic acid, and deep phenol-based methods.(40–46, 38, 39) In this chapter we discuss the use of medium and deep peels for postacne scars treatment.

Trichloroacetic acid (TCA) is the most common chemical used in medium-depth peels. TCA ($C(Cl)_3COOH$) is found as anhydrous hygroscopic crystals. TCA is a strong acid with pK_a of 0.26. Its destructive activity is related to the acidity of the solution; therefore, more concentrated solutions of TCA create more destructive effect on the skin.

The solutions for deep peeling are based on a combination of phenol and croton oil. **Phenol** ($C5H5OH$) or carbolic acid is an aromatic hydrocarbon derived originally from coal tar, but prepared synthetically in a process that utilizes monochlorobenzene as a starting point; 98% phenol appears as transparent crystals, whereas liquefied phenol consists of 88% USP solution of phenol in water.

Other chemicals such as hydroquinone and resorcinol, widely used in cosmetic dermatology, share similar chemical structure with phenol.

Croton oil is an extract of the seed of the plant *Croton tiglium* and has been commercially prepared as Croton resin since 1932. Its activity on the skin is related to free hydroxyl groups that cause skin vesiculation even in low doses.

Other chemicals in use in deep chemical peel formulas include septisol, water, vegetable oils (glycerin, olive, sesame).

All the modern phenol formulas are based and modified from a few lay peelers' formulations. Names such as Grade/, Coopersmith, Kelsen, and Maschek are the origins of Baker-Gordon's, Brown's, Hetter's, Stone's, Litton's, Exoderm, and other formulas. All of them are based on the aforementioned chemical components in different concentrations. Concentration of phenol ranges between 45% and 80%, whereas concentration of croton oil ranges between 0.16% and 2.05%. It is generally accepted that the role of liquid soap is to reduce the skin-surface tension and to improve solution penetration. In spite of this, septisol is not included in all of the formulas. Some of the formulas contain oils. The role of the oils in the formula has not been clarified yet. Our personal experience shows that oily phenol solution penetrates the skin in a slower and controllable fashion.

TECHNOLOGY

1. Medium-depth peels

Trichloroacetic acid is the most common chemical used in medium depth peels. Whereas 10% to 20% TCA creates superficial skin exfoliation, 35% concentration peels the skin down to the upper dermal layers. Concentrations higher than 35% are not recommended because the results are less predictable and the potential for scarring increases significantly. In order to increase the depth and efficacy of TCA peel, without increasing the concentration of the acid, it has been suggested to combine this chemical with Jessner's solution (Monheit method), 70% glycolic acid (Coleman method), or solid CO2 (Brody method).

TCA solution is compounded in a weight to volume preparation. To prepare a 35% solution we dissolve 35 g of TCA crystals in a small amount of water and add water to make a total volume of 100 ml. TCA is stable in room temperature and not light sensitive.

Skin preparation is important before TCA peel performance. This includes retin A (0.25%–0.1%) cream, glycolic acid–based moisturizer, and hydroquinone containing preparation starting 2 to 6 weeks before the procedure. Systemic antiherpertic agent is initiated a day before the peel. Before starting the procedure, all patients are photographed and sign consent form.

Prior to the peeling solution application, a thorough cleaning of the skin is performed with a detergent solution; thereafter, defatting is done using acetone. TCA peel can be performed under intravenous sedation, but in most cases a combination of oral sedative such as lorazepam or diazepam and analgesic, such as tramadol is sufficient.

Cotton q-tips or gauzes are dipped in a small container containing the peeling solution and squeezed properly to avoid dripping of the solution to undesired areas. Using a gauze, more aggressive abrasive effect is achieved. If TCA is painted by a q-tip, more superficial effect is created. In treatment of scarred facial skin, we use both tools alternatively during a single treatment according to the damage severity in each area. Whatever tool is used, TCA solution is applied systematically according to the cosmetic units until white frost appears. The degree of the frosting correlates with the depth of solution penetration. Level I is speckled white frosting with mild erythema and corresponds to superficial penetration. Level II is characterized by an even white-coated frost with background erythema (Figure 6.1). This degree of frosting is usually desirable for medium-depth peels. Level III is solid white opaque frost with little or no background erythema, usually characterizing deep peels and not desirable in TCA procedure.

As frosting develops, cooling of the area using wet, cold compresses provides symptomatic relief of the burning sensation and does not neutralize TCA. A patient usually becomes completely comfortable 15 to 20 minutes after the procedure when all the frosting subsides.

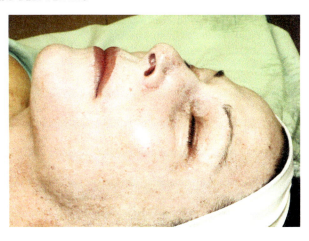

Figure 6.1 Level-II frosting achieved during 35% peel.

After-peel care includes continuous wetting of the skin. During the next days patients may expect to feel tightening and swelling of the skin together with gradual darkening of the skin color. On Day 3 or 4 the skin starts to crack and desquamation begins. At this stage moisturizing cream can be applied. Full reepithelization is completed after 5 to 7 days. At this stage patient is advised to wear comoupflage makeup and resume normal daily activities. Blunt moisturizer and high-level sun protection are recommended for the next 2 to 3 weeks.

The mechanism of action of medium-depth peels includes restoration of keratinocyte polarity and increase in collagen type I content.(47)

Focal application of high-concentration TCA on acne scars has been reported and labeled as chemical reconstruction of skin scars (CROSS).(43, 48) In this technique 95% TCA solution is applied by a sharp applicator into the ice-pick acne scars without affecting adjacent areas. White frosting is achieved shortly. The postpeel course is identical to the full-face procedure. Treatments are repeated every 3 to 6 weeks, up to the total of 6 treatments; 50% TCA can be used locally in the same fashion to treat exfacial acne scars.(49)

2. Combination peels

Combination peels are performed when deeper effect on the skin is required, yet deep peeling is not considered an option.

1. Monheit's combination: (50) Jessner's solution with 35% TCA. Classical Jessner's solution is composed of resorcinol (14%), lactic acid (14%), and salicylic acid (14%) in alcoholic solution, and modified Jessner's contains lactic acid (17%), salicylic acid (17%), and citric acid (8%) in ethanol. After washing the face, peeling solution is applied using wet gauze systematically covering facial cosmetic units. Repeated coats are usually needed until erythema and patchy frost develops. At this stage TCA is applied using q-tip. Some authors recommend to wait 5 minutes between the Jessner's solution

and application of TCA. The after-peel course and care are similar to that of TCA peel.

2. Brody's combination: (51) Icing the skin with solid CO2 deepens the penetration of TCA and improves the clinical effect. Main indications for this combination are flattening the edges of depressed acne scars, actinic and seborrheic keratosis, and fine wrinkles. The depth of the skin icing is determined by the exposure time of the skin to CO2. Usually the skin is rubbed for 5 (mild exposure) to 15 (hard exposure) seconds. The application of TCA is performed in a normal fashion.

3. Coleman's combination: (52) Glycolic acid at 70% is applied usually for 2 minutes and neutralized before further application of TCA. This combination is least likely to produce pigmentation complications.

4. Combination with dermabrasion: To improve efficacy of the procedure, the peel can be combined with mechanical dermabrasion.

3. Deep peels

All patients are required to perform electrocardiogram and complete blood count prior to the procedure. Any heart disease requires special precautions, and it is always recommended to work in cooperation with patient's cardiologist.

Prophylactic acyclovir, valacyclovir, or famvir is given to patients with history of recurrent herpes simplex, starting in a day before the procedure and continuing for 10 days until full reepithelialization is achieved. It is still debatable whether preparation of the skin is required for deep chemical peeling. We feel that topical retin A preparations used daily for 2 to 6 weeks prior to the procedure may create better and more even penetration of the peeling solution in sebaceous and hyperkeratotic skins.

Standard photography and consent form are always obtained before the procedure.

Full-face deep peels should be carried out under full cardiopulmonary monitoring with intravenous hydration throughout the procedure. Intravenous sedation or regional blocks make the procedure pain free. Before the peeling, meticulous degreasing of the skin is performed using oil-free acetone-soaked gauze sponges. This step is imperative to obtain even penetration of the solution into the skin.

For application of the peeling solution hand-made cotton-tipped applicators are employed. The application of phenol solution is accomplished with semidry applicator. The usual end point is ivory-white to gray-white color of skin (Figure 6.2). All the cosmetic units are gradually covered. At this stage we combine mechanical skin dermabrasion by using a tipolisher, which is sterile surgical equipment designed originally for cleaning cauthery tips during operations (Figure 6.3). This simple disposable tool is available in any standard operating setting. Another option is to use sterilized gentle sandpaper. At this stage pin-point bleeding is observed. Reapplication of peeling solution coagulates most of the bleeding. The face is covered with impermeable tape mask for 24 hours (Figure 6.4). After

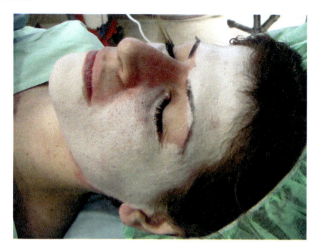

Figure 6.2 The application of phenol solution creates ivory-white to gray-white color of skin.

24 hours, the tape mask is removed and the exudate is cleansed with sterile saline. Regional reapplication of peeling solution and retaping of the scarred areas is performed and the tape is left for an additional 4 to 6 hours and then removed by the patient. The face is covered with bismuth subgalate antiseptic powder for 7 days (Figure 6.5). On the Day 8, wet soaking with tap water while standing in the shower is used to soften the powder mask and to remove it. The erythema gradually subsides over 2 months. During this time, makeup with a green foundation is encouraged to use that assists the patient to resume all the daily activities. The third phase of the treatment is regional repeeling, being performed 6 to 8 weeks after the original treatment. This phase is optional for patients with residual scar areas.(39)

COMPLICATIONS

The list of potential complications of chemical peels includes pigmentary changes, infections, milia, acneform eruption, scarring, and cardiotoxicity.

1. Pigmentary changes—reactive hyperpigmentation can occur after any depth of chemical peels. Usually lighter complexions have lower risk for hyperpigmentation, but genetic factors play an important role, and sometimes light patients with "dark genes" hyperpigment unexpectedly. Skin priming using a combination of hydroquinone and tretinoin cream (Kligman's formulation) before the medium-depth peels, and early introduction of this preparation after deep peels, reduces the rate of this complication. Demarcation lines can be avoided if the boundaries of the peeling area are hidden under the mandibular line and feathered gradually to the normal skin. Hypopigmentation after phenol peels is proportional to the depth of the peel, amount of the solution used, numbers of drops of crotton oil in the solution, inherent skin color, and postpeel sun-related

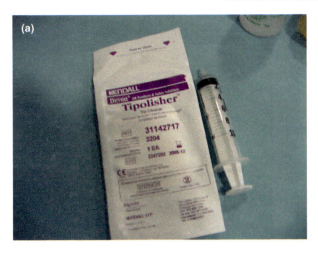
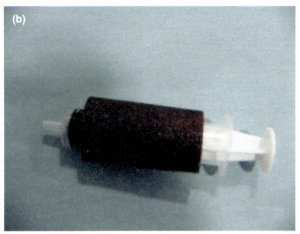

Figure 6.3 (A) Tipolisher is sterile surgical equipment designed originally for cleaning cauthery tips during operations. (B) Tipolisher is attached to standard 10-ml syringe to perform skin abrasion.

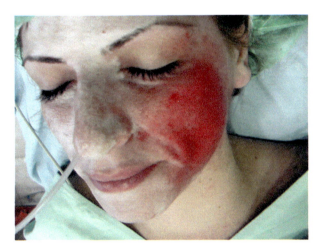

Figure 6.4 Bleeding is observed following skin abrasion using tipolosher.

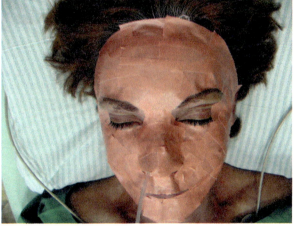

Figure 6.5 The face is covered with impermeable tape mask for 24 hours.

behavior. Hypopigmentation is a major drawback for performing medium and deep peels focally. Intradermal nevi can hyperpigment after deep peels.

2. Infection—bacterial and fungal complications in chemical peels are rare. Patients with positive history of herpes simplex infection are treated prophylactically with acyclovir or valacyclovir during medium and deep peel until full reepithelization is achieved. Toxic-shock syndrome has been reported after chemical peel.(53)

3. Milia or epidermal cysts appear in up to 20% of patients after chemical peels, usually 8 to 16 weeks after the procedure. Electrosurgery is simple and effective to treat this post peel complication.

4. Acneiform dermatitis—acneiform eruption after chemical peels is not rare and usually appears immediately after reepithelialization. Its etiology is multifactorial and is related to either exacerbation of previously existing acne or is due to overgreasing of newly formed skin. This complication is not uncommon when treating thick sebaceous skin complexions, which is frequently the case in acne-scarred patients. Short-term systemic antibiotics together with discontinuation of any oily preparations will usually provide satisfactory. If not effective enough, short course of oral isotretinoin will be usually satiscfactory.

5. Scarring—scarring remains to be the most dreadful complication of chemical peels. The contributing factors are not well understood yet. The most common location of the scars is in the lower part of the face, probably due to more aggressive treatment in this area or due to the greater tissue movement or due to eating and speaking during the

healing process. Delayed healing and persistent redness are important alarming signs for forthcoming scarring. Topical antibiotics and potent steroid preparations should be introduced as soon as this diagnosis is made.

6. The most important potential complication exclusive to phenol-based peels is cardiotoxicity. Phenol is directly toxic to myocardium. Studies in rats showed decrease in myocardial contraction and in electrical activity following systemic exposure to phenol.(54) Since fatal doses ranged widely in these studies it seems that individual sensitivity of myocardium to this chemical exists. In humans sex, age, previous cardiac history, or blood phenol levels are not accurate predictors for cardiac arrhythmia susceptibility. (55) Cardiac arrhythmias have been recorded in up to 23% of patients when full-face peel was performed in less than 30 minutes.(56) Adequate patient's management reduces this complication to less than 7%.(57) No hepatorenal or central nervous system toxicities have been reported in the literature with properly performed chemical peels.

OUTLOOK AND FUTURE DEVELOPMENTS

In spite of the high level of improvement achieved using chemical peels, acne scars are still challenging, especially in young individuals. In most cases, a complete smoothening of the skin is impossible, especially on the tight skin areas, such a forehead and temples. This is an essential message to be clearly conveyed to a patient before the intervention to build up an appropriate level of expectations. Patients have to be shown pre- and post-treatment photographs and to be asked about their expectations (Figure 6.6, 6.7). All exaggerated expectations should be

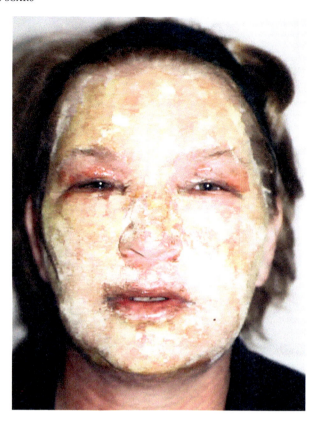

Figure 6.6 The face is covered with bismuth subgalate antiseptic powder for 7 days.

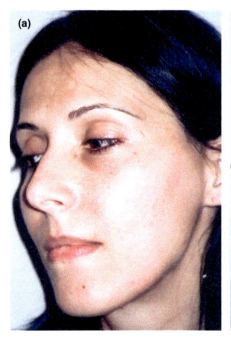
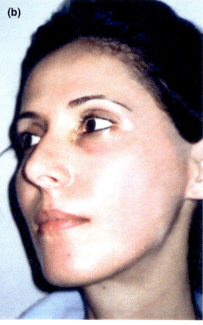

Figure 6.7 A 32-year-old woman: (A) before and (B) 4 weeks after deep peeling (Exoderm method) combined with mechanical dermabrasion.

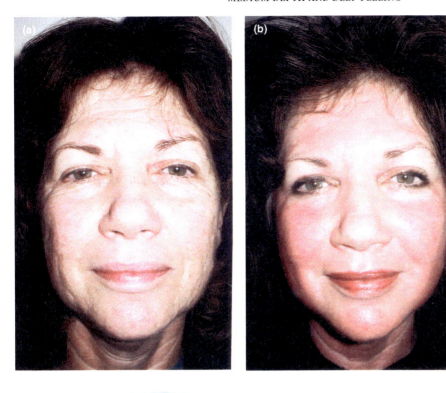

Figure 6.8 A 56-year-old fair-skinned woman: (A) before and (B) 2 weeks after deep peeling combined with dermabrasion.

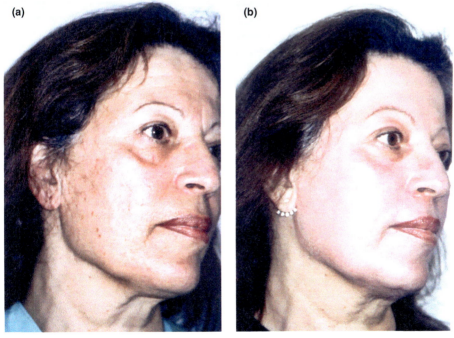

Figure 6.9 A 62-year-old dark-skinned woman: (A) before and (B) 4 weeks after deep peeling combined with dermabrasion.

discouraged. A need for repeating peeling sessions, limited to the most scarred areas, is also discussed.

In general, best results are achieved in older female patients, rather than in young males (Figures 6.8 and 6.9). Atrophic scars response better than ice-picked and hypertrophic ones. Deeper the procedure, more significant the result achieved. Therefore, while with phenol-based peel a single or double treatment is required, TCA-treated patients are expected to have multiple sessions.

Nonfacial skin is a special challenge. Because healing process is less effective in this skin, only milder peels are possible to be performed. Therefore, the results are usually less adequate.

In my opinion, future development will include a combination of chemical abrasion of the facial skin with topical application of fractional ablative or nonablative light technologies. Though promising, these technologies per se have not yet provided comparable results to chemical peels. With time, the appropriate combination will be found.

REFERENCES

1. Baker TM. Chemical and lasers for skin resurfacing. Aesthetic Surg 1999; 19: 325–7.
2. Landau M. Chemical peels. Clin Dermatol 2008; 26: 200–8.
3. Burton JL, Cunliffe WJ, Stafford I, Shuster S. The prevalence of acne vulgaris in adolescence. Br J Dermatol 1971; 85: 119–26.
4. Rademaker M, Garioch JJ, Simpson NB. Acne in school-children: no longer a concern for dermatologists. BMJ 1989; 298: 1217–9.
5. Cunliffe3 WJ, Gould DJ. Prevalence of facial acne vulgaris in late adolescence and in adults. BMJ 1979; 1: 1109–10.
6. Layton AM, Henderson CA, Cunliffe WJ. A clinical evaluation of acne scarring and its incidence. Clin Exp Dermatol 1994; 19: 303–8.
7. Holland DB, Jeremy AHT, Roberts SG, Seukeran DC, Layton AM. Inflammation in acne scarring: a comparison of the responses inlesions from patients prone and not prone to scar. Br J Dermatol 2004; 150: 72–81.
8. Mackee GM, Karp FL. The treatment of post acne scars with phenol. Br J Dermatol 1952; 64: 456–9.
9. Kurtin A. Corrective surgical planing of skin: new technique for treatment of acne scars and other skin defects. AMA Arch Derm Syphilol 1953; 68: 389–97.
10. Malherbe WD, Davies DS. Surgical treatment of acne scarring, by a dermatome. Plast Reconstr Surg 1971; 47: 122–6.
11. Orentreich N. Dermabrasion. J Am Med Womens Assoc 1969; 24: 331–6.
12. Kurtin A. Dermabrasion. Arch Dermatol 1968; 98: 87.
13. Rattner R, Rein CR. Treatment of acne scars by dermabrasion; rotary brush method. J Am Med Assoc 1955; 159: 1299–301.
14. Knapp TR, Kaplan EN, Danieks JR. Injectable collagen for soft tissue augmentation. Plast Reconstr Surg 1977; 60: 398–405.
15. Stegman SJ, Tromovitch TA. Implantation of collagen for depressed scars. J Dermatol Surg Oncol 1980; 6: 450–3.
16. Varnavides CK, Forster RA, Cunliffe WJ. The role of bovine collagen in the treatment of acne scars. Br J Dermatol 1987; 116: 199–206.
17. Thrimbke JR. Dermal overgarfting in dermatology. J Dermatol Surg Oncol 1983; 9: 987–93.
18. Dzubow LM. Scar revision by punch-graft transplants. J Dermatol Surg Oncol 1985; 11: 1200–2.
19. BeseckerB, Hart CG. A new treatment option for acne scars: allograft dermis. Dermatol Nurs 1999; 11: 111–4.
20. Goodman G. Laser-assisted dermal grafting for the correction of cutaneous contour defects. Dermatol Surg 1997; 23: 95–9.
21. Mancuso A, Farber GA. The abraded punch graft for pitted facial scars. J Dermatol Surg Oncol 1991; 17: 32–4.
22. Sulamanidze MA, Salti G, Mascceti M, Sulamanidze GM. Wire scalpel for surgical correction of soft tissue contour defects by subcutaneous dissection. Dermatol Surg 2000; 26: 146–50.
23. Garrett AB, Dufresne RG Jr, Ratz JL, Berlin AJ. Carbon dioxide laser treatment of pitted acne scarring. J Dermatol Surg Oncol 1990; 16: 737–40.
24. Alster TS, West TB. Resurfacing of atrophic facial acne scars with a high-energy, pulsed carbon dioxide laser. Dermatol Surg 1996; 22; 151–4.
25. Alster TS, McMeekin TO. Improvement of facial acne scars by the 585 nm flashlamp-pumped pulsed dye laser. J Am Acad Dermatol 1996; 35: 79–81.
26. Kye YC. Resurfacing of pitted facial scars with a pulsed Er:YAG laser. Dermatol Surg 1997; 23: 880–3.
27. West TB. Laser resurfacing of atrophic scars. Dermatol Clin 1997; 15: 449–57.
28. Manusciatti W, Fitzpatrick RE, Goldman MP. Treatment of facial skin using combinations of CO2, Q-switched alexandrite, flashlamp-pumped pulsed dye, and Er:YAG lasers in the same treatment session. Dermatol Surg 2000; 26: 114–20.
29. Jordan R, Cummins C, Burls A. Laser resurfacing of the skin for the improvement of facial acne scarring: a systematic review of the evidence. Br J Dermatol 2000; 142: 413–23.
30. Tsai RY, Wang CN, Chan HL. Aluminum oxide crystal microdermabrasion. A new technique for treating facial scarring. Dermatol Surg 1995; 21: 539–42.
31. Goodman GJ. Post acne scarring: a review. J Cosmet Laser Ther 2003; 5: 77–95.
32. Fulton JE Jr. Modern dermabrasion techniques: a personal appraisal. J Dermatol Surg Oncol 1987; 13: 780–9.
33. Solotoff SA. Treatment for pitted acne scarring–postauricular punch grafts followed by dermabrasion. J Dermatol Surg Oncol 1986; 12: 1079–84.
34. Grevelink JM, White VR. Concurrent use of laser skin resurfacing and punch excision in the treatment of facial acne scarring. Dermatol Surg 1998; 24: 527–30.
35. Fulton JE Jr. Dermabrasion, chemabrasion, and laserabrasion. Historical perspectives, modern dermabrasion techniques, and future trends. Dermatol Surg 1996; 22: 619–28.
36. Ayhan S, Baran CN, Yavuzer R et al. Combined chemical peeling and dermabrasion for deep acne and posttraumatic scars as well as aging face. Plast Reconstr Surg 1998; 102(4): 1238–46.

37. Horton CE, Sadove RC. Refinements in combined chemical peel and simultaneous abrasion of the face. Ann Plast Surg 1987; 19(6): 504–11.

38. Fintsi Y, Kaplan H, Landau M. Whether to peel or laser for acne scarring and hyperpigmentation. Int J Cosm Surg 1999; 7: 67–70.

39. Fintsi Y. Exoderm chemabrasion: original method for the treatment of facial acne scars. Int J Cosm Surg 1998; 6: 111–4.

40. Atzori L, Brundu MA, Orru A, Biggio P. Glycolic acid peeling in the treatment of acne. J Eur Acad Dermatol Venereol 1999; 12: 119–22.

41. Jansen T. Chemical peeling. Impressive results in acne scars and aging skin. MMW Fortschr Med 2000; 142: 39–41.

42. Al-Waiz MM, Al-Sharqi AI. Medium-depth chemical peels in the treatment of acne scars in dark-skinned individuals. Dermatol Surg 2002; 28: 383–7.

43. Lee JB, Chung WG, Kwahck H, Lee KH. Focal treatment of acne scars with trichloroacetic acid: chemical reconstruction of skin scars method. Dermatol Surg 2002; 28: 1017–21.

44. Wang KK, Lee M. The principle of a three-staged operation in the surgery of acne scars. J Am Acad Dermatol 1999; 40: 95–7.

45. Park JH, Choi YD, Kim SW, Kim YC, Park SW. Effectiveness of modified phenol peel (Exoderm) on facial wrinkles, acne scars and other skin problems of Asian patients. J Dermatol 2007; 34: 17–24.

46. Swinehart JM. Case reports: surgical therapy of acne scars in pigmented skin. J Drugs Dermatol 2007; 6: 74–7.

47. Nelson BR, Fader DJ, Gillard M, Majmudar G, Johnson TM. Pilot histologic and ultrastructural study of the effects of medium-depth chemical facial peels on dermal collagen in patients with actinically damaged skin. J Am Acad Dermatol 1995; 32: 472–8.

48. Yug A, Lane JE, Howard MS, Kent DE. Histologic study of depressed acne scars treated with serial high-concentration (95%) trichloroacetic acid. Dermatol Surg 2006; 32(8): 985–90.

49. Fabbrocini G, Cacciapuotu S, Fardella N, Pastore F, Monfrecola G. CROSS technique: chemical reconstruction of skin scars method. Dermatol Ther 2008; 21(Suppl 3): S29–32.

50. Monheit GD. The Jessner's-trichloroacetic acid peel. An enhanced medium-depth chemical peel. Dermatol Clin 1995; 13: 277–83.

51. Brody HJ, Hailey CW. Medium-depth chemical peeling of the skin: a variation of superficial chemosurgery. J Dermatol Surg Oncol 1986; 12: 1268–75.

52. Coleman WP 3rd, Futrell JM. The glycolic acid trichloroacetic acid peel. J Dermatol Surg Oncol 1994; 20: 76–80.

53. Holm C, Muhlbauer W. Toxic shock syndrome in plastic surgery patients: case report and review of the literature. Aesthetic Plast Surg 1998; 22: 180–4.

54. Stagnone GJ, Orgel MB, Stagnone JJ. Cardiovascular effects of topical 50% trichloroacetic acid and Baker's phenol solution. J Dermatol Surg Oncol 1987; 13: 999–1002.

55. Litton C, Trinidad G. Complications of chemical face peeling as evaluated by a questionnaire. Plast Reconstr Surg 1981; 67: 738–44.

56. Truppman F, Ellenbery J. The major electrocardiographic changes during chemical face peeling. Plast Reconstr Surg 1979; 63: 44.

57. Landau M. Cardiac complications in deep chemical peels. Dermatol Surg 2007; 33: 190–3.

7 Dermabrasion for acne scars
Christopher B Harmon and Jens J Thiele

KEY FEATURES

- Dermabrasion is one of the most effective therapies for acne scars
- Dermabrasion involves mechanically removing the epidermis and papillary dermis, creating a newly contoured open wound to heal by second intention
- Reepithelialization of dermabraded skin occurs by upward migration of cells from the adnexal structures including hair follicles, sebaceous glands, and sweat ducts.
- Patient selection is key to obtaining excellent results.
- Patients must have realistic expectations of the anticipated improvement, possible side effects, and potential complications of dermabrasion prior to treatment.
- A familiarity with perioperative care and proper operative technique is instrumental to optimal cosmetic outcomes.

INTRODUCTION

Acne vulgaris affects most people at some time in their life. This common condition can have devastating effects on a person's quality of life and may leave permanent scars.(1) Acne scarring is common but surprisingly difficult to treat. Scars can involve textural change in the superficial and deep dermis and can also be associated with erythema, and less often, pigmentary change.(2) Dermabrasion is a skin-resurfacing technique that surgically abrades or planes the epidermis and papillary dermis by contact with an abrasive surface. The latter can be operated either manually (Dermasanding) or motorized, using a rapidly rotating wire brush or diamond fraise.(3) Since the mid-1950s, dermabrasion has been the treatment of choice for resurfacing deep facial scars induced by surgery, trauma, chicken pox, or acne. Dermabrasion is a technique that allows the physician to sculpt the skin surface by surgically abrading, or planning the contours of the skin.(4) User technique, device settings, and the combination of dermabrasion with other skin-resurfacing treatments enable the physician to treat a wide variety of skin defects. With the advent of ablative and nonablative lasers, there has been a great resurgence of resurfacing treatments. Newer modalities using the principles of fractional photothermolysis create patterns of tiny microscopic wounds surrounded by undamaged tissue beneath the skin with an erbium-doped 1,550 nm laser. These devices produce more modest results in many cases than traditional carbon dioxide (CO_2) lasers but with fewer side effects and shorter recovery periods.(5) The limitation of laser resurfacing, however, lies in the unwanted scarring and erythema that can result from excessive thermal injury.

Dermabrasion is a resurfacing technique for deep defects of the skin without the risk for thermal injury.

HISTORY

In its simplest form, dermabrasion was used by ancient Egyptians in circa 1500 B.C., who employed the abrasive characteristics of pumice and alabaster to treat skin blemishes.(6, 7) In 1905, the German dermatologist Kromayer first reported controlled abrasion of the skin.(8) His technique involved the use of rotating wheels and rasps, which differed little from tools used for present-day dermabrasion. He treated acne scars, keratoses, and areas of hyperpigmentation. Despite this early report of surgical planing, dermabrasion did not gain widespread popularity until the early 1950s.(6) Since the mid-1950s, growing interest in the technique has culminated in its application to a variety of lesions and has more recently expanded to include facial scars secondary to acne, trauma, surgery, and varicella zoster virus. The growing number of applications of dermabrasion has been accompanied by evolution of the technique from the use of common sandpaper in the mid-20th century to electrically powered devices with wire-brush tips or diamond fraises of varying sizes, shapes, and textures that can achieve speeds of over 33,000 revolutions per minute.(7) The most aggressive abrading end piece is the wire brush, a 3.0 × 17.0 mm wheel with bristles radiating from the center. While the wire brush can be technically difficult to master, its microlacerations are the most efficient means of removing the nodules of rhinophyma, the thick plaques of hypertrophic scars, or deep acne scars. As a technique, dermabrasion has become the gold standard for resurfacing and is, at present, the comparator against which all other means of resurfacing are evaluated.

BASIC SCIENCE

Resurfacing, by definition, involves iatrogenic removal of one or multiple layers of the skin to create a cutaneous wound. Dermabrasion mechanically removes the epidermis and papillary dermis, creating a partial thickness wound to heal by second intention.(4) In partial-thickness wounds, because the deep dermis has not been lost or destroyed, adnexal structures are present. These structures serve as a reservoir of epithelial cells for repopulating the epidermis. Epithelia from these structures, as well as from the ulcer edge, migrate across the wound surface to provide coverage. This well-characterized, yet complex, wound healing response is triggered involving transforming growth factor beta (TGF-β)–driven myofibroblastic deposition of new Type I and Type III collagen and subsequent remodelling in the dermis. In addition, TGF-β, keratinocyte growth factor (KGF), and epidermal growth factor (EGF) stimulate reepithelialization from both underlying skin appendages and adjacent epithelialized skin.(9)

Defined ultrastructural and molecular alterations accompany the clinically visible changes apparent in the dermabraded area. These include increased collagen-bundle density and size with a tendency toward unidirectional orientation of collagen fibers parallel to the epidermal surface, as well as altered levels of $\alpha6$- and $\beta4$-integrin expression in the stratum spinosum and changes in the distribution of tenascin expression.(10) Dermabrasive modification of the extracellular ligand expression of the primary cicatrix influences epithelial cell-to-cell interactions and reorganization of the underlying connective tissue, thereby producing a less perceptible scar.(3)

INDICATIONS

The type of scarring seen usually dictates which treatment modality will be the most effective.(11) Scars are typically visible to the observer if they are abnormally colored or shaped, have an altered contour or textures, or are longer than about 1 cm in length.(12) Currently, there is no universally accepted classification of acne scarring. Jacob et al. proposed a three-term system: "ice-pick", "rolling" and "boxcar" scars. Ice-pick scars are described as narrow, deep, sharply demarcated tracts that extend vertically into deep dermis or subcutaneous layer. Rolling scars occur from dermal tethering of otherwise relatively normal-looking skin. They are usually wider than 4 to 5 mm. 'Boxcar scars' are small-diameter, shallow lesions (Figure 7.1A–E).(13)

With regard to acne scarring, even in the era of laser devices, fractionated delivery approaches and noninvasive "tissue-tightening" procedures, dermabrasion remains an important tool in the combination approach to the improvement of acne scarring. Whereas the shallow and wide, undulating, or "rolling" type acne scars are better treated with subcision, dermal grafts, fillers, or fractionated laser devices, the slightly deeper and narrower "boxcar" type acne scars that demonstrate step-off vertical borders respond best to mechanical dermabrasion.(11) In addition, the deepest and narrowest "ice-pick" type acne scars respond best to dermabrasion subsequent to punch excisions, punch grafts, or TCA cross destruction. 'Rolling' scars are large-diameter, atrophic, distensible, or bound-down scars that may require subcision (14) to release tethering scar tissue and thicken the dermis through fibroplasia. As a complement to the use of injectable fillers, dermabrasion can produce significant improvement in rolling acne scars as well.(4)

ADVANTAGES AND DISADVANTAGES

As compared to fully ablative resurfacing with the CO_2 and Er:YAG lasers, dermabrasion demonstrates similar or greater efficacy for the treatment of scars, with less postoperative erythema and more rapid reepithelialization. Though newer, fractionated delivery protocols result in even less erythema and quicker reepithelialization than dermabrasion [Chapas, 2008 #34], their efficacies for the improvement of scars rarely match that seen with mechanical dermabrasion.

The major disadvantage of dermabrasion as compared to the above modalities is that it is much more operator dependent. Unlike laser and light devices, the depth of penetration is not preprogrammed. Successful treatment relies not only on the physician's knowledge of the modality and application settings but also on his or her skilled execution.[Spencer, 2005 #17] In the novice's hands, dermabrasion exhibits a narrower window or buffer between effective treatment depth and inappropriate scarring depth. While resurfacing of the epidermis and upper dermis is desired, accidental injury of deeper reticular dermis results in full thickness wounds and thus additional scarring. However, this method is usually quickly learned by dermatologists trained by experienced Dermasurgeons

PREOPERATIVE CONSIDERATIONS

Appropriate patient selection is key to obtaining excellent results. The risk/benefit ratio of dermabrasion in patients who are immunosuppressed or have a history of koebnerizing conditions such as lichen planus or psoriasis, a propensity toward hyper- or hypo-pigmentation, or hypertrophic scar/keloid formation may not be favorable. Similarly, in patients who have undergone a prior procedure involving the area to be dermabraded, for example, surgical excision, grafting, or other procedures requiring extensive undermining, at least 6 to 8 weeks should elapse before dermabrasion is considered, and many surgeons prefer to wait 6 months or more after a face lift before dermabrading.

Because dermabrasion produces aerosolized particles, preoperative planning should begin with HIV testing and a hepatitis panel. A thorough past medical history including prior and present acne regimens is also a necessary part of the preoperative workup for dermabrasion, and a recent history of isotretinoin use is a contraindication to dermabrasion because this combination has been linked to the development of hypertrophic scars.(15) As a general rule, 6 months is considered an adequate interval between cessation of isotretinoin use and dermabrasion. A short (2–3 week) preoperative course of tretinoin cream has the benefit of reducing the time required for reepithelialization after dermabrasion, and patients with Fitzpatrick type III or IV skin should be treated with a 2- to 4-week preoperative course of hydroquinone cream at 4% to minimize the risk of postoperative hyperpigmentation. Prophylactic antibiotics (cephalexin, 1 to 2 gm daily for 10 to 14 days) should be given only to patients with a history of impetigo but are otherwise not required. In contrast, the potential risk of herpes virus reactivation necessitates that all patients be treated with prophylactic antiviral medications (valacyclovir 1 gm daily or famciclovir 500 mg daily), and prophylaxis should continue until full reepithelialization has occurred, or for 14 days after the procedure. Full-face dermabrasion requires oral or intramuscular sedation in conjunction with the use of cryoanesthesia, local or tumescent anesthesia, and nerve blocks. Meperidine hydrochloride

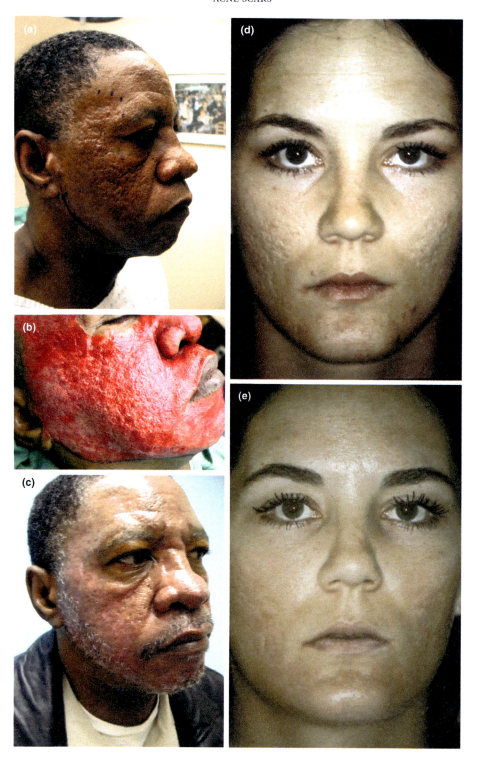

Figure 7.1 (A–E) Dermabrasion of acne scars. (A) Severe acne scarring present in an African American male prior to dermabrasion. (B) Postoperative appearance of the treated area. (C) Appearance of the treated area 4 weeks after dermabrasion. (D) Moderately severe acne scarring present in a Caucasian female. (E) Appearance of the treated area 12 weeks after dermabrasion.

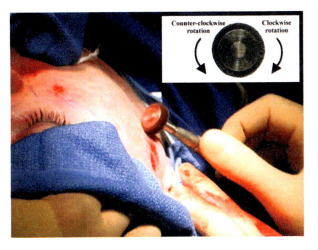

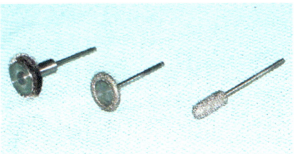

Figure 7.3 Endpieces commonly used in dermabrasion. From left to right, wire brush, diamond fraize and cone-shaped diamond fraize.

Figure 7.2 Photograph demonstrating correct hand position of the operator on the dermabrasion hand piece Arciform strokes are performed by pulling the hand engine perpendicular to the direction of the rotating endpiece. *Insert in right upper corner* depicts the wire-brush abrading wheel with steel bristles radiating from the center in a clockwise fashion. Counterclockwise rotation offers a less aggressive approach.

75 mg i.m. can be given with 25 mg of i.m. hydroxyzine 30 to 60 minutes prior to placement of central nerve blocks and tumescent anesthesia, and 5 to 10 mg of diazepam can be given sublingually to reduce intraoperative anxiety. Prior to anesthetization, the operative area should be cleansed with chlorhexidine 4% solution. Central nerve blocks of the supratrochlear, supraorbital, infraorbital, and mental nerves provide adequate anesthesia of the central face. The perinasal ring block anesthetizes the nose, and the infiltration of the lateral cheeks with 150 to 250 cc of 0.25% tumescent lidocaine solution delivered through a 25-gauge spinal needle advanced medially from a preauricular insertion point provides sufficient anesthesia for both superficial and deep abrasions in an office-based setting. (16) Preoperative application of petroleum jelly, aquaphor, or K-Y jelly along the hair line minimizes entanglement of the hair with the spinning tip of the hand engine.

TECHNICAL PROCEDURE

Whether abrading acne scars or surgical scars, the technique is similar. The hand engine (Bell, Osada, Permark) is held with the four fingers of the hand, and the neck of the engine is stabilized with the thumb (Figure 7.2). Refrigerant spray (Frigiderm, containing Freon 114) is not required in every case but can be a useful adjunct when treating large thick scars. It should be applied to the treatment area followed by a 5- to 10-second thaw time, provides some anesthesia, and most importantly, freezes the deeper and thicker scars so that they become a solid substrate upon which the shoulders of the scar can be recontoured. Scars should be frozen without stretching,

as this preserves the relaxed natural state of the scar and allows for better visualization of the fine textural detail. Once the scar is frozen, three-point retraction is accomplished by the two hands of the surgical assistant and the nondominant hand of the surgeon. Passes over the treatment area are made with unidirectional strokes perpendicular to the direction of the rotating wire brush (Figure 7.2). Regarding dermabrasion with the wire brush, the direction of end-piece rotation, with or against the angle of the radiating bristles, controls the thickness of the tissue plane removed with each pass. Consequently, thicker scars are more efficiently treated with the wire-brush (Figure 7.3) rotating in a clockwise (against the angle of the radiating bristles) direction, and counter-clockwise (with the angle of the radiating bristles) rotation offers a less aggressive approach (Figure 7.2, insert). With the wire brush and the coarse diamond fraise, red papillary dots of bleeding herald entry into the papillary dermis. The bleeding foci become larger and admixed with frayed collagen debris upon entry into the reticular dermis. Scars frequently crumble or disintegrate upon abrasion, which provides another visual endpoint for performing this resurfacing surgery. The boundaries of the abraded area should be feathered in order to avoid step-off lesions or drastic pigment changes. Typically, treatment zones are designed along the borders of cosmetic subunits for spot dermabrasion or 1 to 2 cm below the mandible for full-face dermabrasion. For full-face dermabrasion, dependent regions of the face, for example, the mandible and the lateral cheeks, should be treated first, as visualization of these areas is the first to become obfuscated by blood and debris. The nose and central face are generally treated last. Cotton towels rather than gauze pads should be used for blotting and retracting, as the latter can become easily entangled in the rapidly rotating tip.

POSTTREATMENT CARE

After completion of a full-face dermabrasion, the application of gauze soaked in 1% lidocaine with epinephrine (1:100,000) under prechilled ice packs helps to achieve hemostasis and soothes postoperative stinging. Triamcinolone acetonide 40 mg i.m. given immediately postoperatively reduces edema in the treated area, and 1 to 2 tablets of propoxyphene N-100 every 4 to 6 hours helps to control postoperative pain. The abraded area is then covered with a semipermeable dressing (Vigilon, C.R. Bard, Inc., Covington, GA; 2nd Skin, Spenco Medical Corp., Waco, TX), nonadherent pads paper tape, gauze, and Surgilast netting (Western Medical Ltd., Tenafly, NJ). The use of semipermeable dressings reduces the time for reepithelialization by up to 40% compared to open techniques of wound care, and this effect is attributed to the ability of these dressings to maintain a critical plane of humidity for epithelial cell migration.(17)

MANAGEMENT OF COMPLICATIONS
The most common complications encountered after dermabrasion are milia and acne flares. Acne flares from the occlusive nature of postoperative dressings can be managed with oral antibiotics, and routine topical acne medications are well tolerated 2 weeks after dermabrasion. Milia formation is a common postoperative sequela following dermabrasion and is treated with gentle extraction after a sturdy epithelium has formed.(18)

Infection, pigment alteration, and scarring are the more portentous complications that may be encountered after dermabrasion. Vigilance in the immediate postoperative period is necessary to identify these complications at an early stage and institute appropriate treatment. Postoperative infections caused by bacteria and fungi present as painful nonhealing erosions, and while relatively uncommon, they can be further minimized by daily dressing changes with careful debridement. If infection is suspected, therapy should be initiated with empiric antibiotics and subsequent culture and sensitivity should be used to guide therapy. The appearance of herpetic lesions should prompt a dose increase of valacyclovir or famciclovir from the prophylactic dose of 1 gm and 500 mg daily to 1 gm and 500 mg 3 times daily, respectively. The presence of bright erythema after the first 2 to 3 postoperative weeks is the first sign of early scar formation and should be treated initially with topical high-potency steroid ointment or Cordran tape (Aqua Pharmaceuticals, LLC, Malvern, PA) and followed every 1 to 2 weeks. Intralesional triamcinolone acetonide (5–40 mg/cc) should be considered with any sign of hypertrophy, induration, or elevation of the treated area. Insufficient response to topical or intralesional corticosteroids may indicate the need for intervention with a pulsed dye laser, which can decrease scar induration and erythema.(19) Postoperative erythema that ensues after complete reepithelialization normally fades completely within 2 to 3 months and green- and yellow-based foundations are well suited for camouflaging this transient condition. Patients are counseled to strictly avoid sun until the postoperative erythema has resolved. In spite of complete postoperative sun avoidance, however, some individuals may show signs of hyperpigmentation over the malar prominences and jaw line. In this case, therapeutic bleaching regimens consisting of topical hydroquinone and tretinoin creams applied once or twice

daily to affected areas are well tolerated and may be started 3 to 4 weeks after dermabrasion. The bleaching regimen should be continued for 4 to 8 weeks after the hyperpigmentation resolves. Permanent hypopigmentation is seen in 20% to 30% of patients and is more common in individuals with Fitzpatrick types III and IV skin. While the mechanism of this condition is incompletely understood, a subset of patients have been shown to respond to treatment with the 308 nm excimer laser.(20) A similar condition called pseudohypopigmentation is seen when normally repigmented abraded skin has a slightly lighter tone and appearance than that of adjacent sun-damaged nonabraded skin. The disparity in skin tones can be reduced with superficial- or medium-depth chemical peels, nonablative lasers, and intense pulsed light to blend the treated and untreated areas. Patients should also be counseled to avoid strenuous exercise for at least 6 weeks because this helps to minimize petechiae in the treated area.

OTHER TECHNIQUES

Manual Dermabrasion
Manual dermabrasion ("dermasanding") involves abrading the underlying skin by hand using silicon carbide sandpaper. Wounding depth depends on the type of paper used, the force applied by the surgeon, and the duration of contact with the skin. Although it can be used to produce a wound as deep as with motorized wire-brush dermabrasion, manual dermasanding is most commonly used as a more superficial resurfacing modality.(21) Since manual dermasanding is so labor intensive, it is rarely used to treat the entire face but rather for resurfacing of localized regions to minimize the appearance of smaller, well-circumscribed scar areas.(22) For treatment of moderate-to-severe acne scarring involving larger areas of the face, the previously described motorized dermabrasion technique remains the gold standard.(21)

Microdermabrasion
Microdermabrasion is the second most widely performed cosmetic procedure in the United States and is commonly offered at spas and beauty salons.(18) The first report on microdermabrasion in the medical literature appeared in 1995 by Tsai et al.(23) Since then, microdermabrasion has been frequently used for a variety of indications including dyschromias, photodamage, acne, and scars. Similar to dermabrasion, microdermabrasion causes direct mechanical skin removal, however, at much more superficial levels. Therefore, it is usually a painless procedure with more texture benefit than permanent surface changes.(24) Often referred to as a "lunch-time" procedure, microdermabrasion has become a popular procedure that is classified as light or very superficial dermabrasion. This method employs aluminum oxide crystals that are propelled at the skin with a pressurized application and vacuum system. The most improvement is achieved with fine wrinkles and postinflammatory hyperpigmentation.

Although not scientifically proven to improve the appearance of scars, many patients report that their skin feels smoother. It is used to treat acne and the hyperpigmentation caused by acne. Despite its widespread use, little is known about its actual mechanism of action. The few published studies suggest that patients and physicians alike report a mild benefit when microdermabrasion is utilized for photoaging. Histological evaluation reveals little actual abrasion of the skin with the procedure, yet changes were reported in the dermis.(25) An increase in epidermal and dermal thickness, flattening of the rete pegs, vascular ectasia with perivascular inflammation, papillary dermal hyalinization, and newly deposited collagen and elastic fibers have all been described.(26) While it is still unclear how dermal remodeling actually occurs, there is some experimental evidence that elevation of transcription factors, primary cytokines, and matrix metalloproteinases occurs rapidly after a single microdermabrasion treatment.(27) Although the thickness of the stratum corneum appears to be unaffected, some studies have shown that microdermabrasion leads to significant alteration in the epidermal barrier function.(28) Thus, microdermabrasion may increase transdermal drug delivery (29) and has been shown to enhance the penetration of topically applied drugs and cosmeceuticals, such as 5-aminolevulinic acid, 5 fluorouracil (23, 30), and antioxidants.(31, 32) Given the safety, simplicity, painlessness, quick recovery time, and relative patient satisfaction associated with microdermabrasion, it is likely to remain a popular treatment. However, to effectively treat the acne-associated facial discoloration, up to 15 treatments may be necessary, which can be very expensive.(33) While most often aluminum oxide crystals are used, occasionally sodium chloride, sodium bicarbonate, or magnesium oxide crystals have been tried in microdermabrasion devices. Newer devices now are crystal free, employing diamond-tipped abrasive devices. Although cheaper, these crystal alternatives are not as abrasive and are less efficacious.(34) Side effects typically include temporary striping of the treatment area; bruising, burning, or stinging sensation; photosensitivity and occasional pain. There is no wounding expected with the force, suction, and speed determining the ultimate depth attained. If using isotretinoin, it is common to wait up to 6 months after the last application to minimize the probability of side effects.(24)

Outlook

Dermabrasion continues to be the technique best supported by the literature and surgical experience for acne scar revision (6) and remains the gold standard to which other resurfacing modalities are compared. It remains to be established whether the emerging laser modalities using the principles of fractional photothermolysis will provide similar or superior results and whether they offer synergistic effects when combined with traditional dermabrasion. As such, future research efforts will continue to refine the technique of dermabrasion, which will undoubtedly remain an extremely valuable tool in our resurfacing armamentarium.(4)

SUMMARY FOR THE CLINICIAN

In the hands of the skilled practitioner, dermabrasion of acne scars can produce excellent results. In general, the indications for dermabrasion include those lesions or skin defects of the epidermis, papillary dermis, and upper reticular dermis that can be partially or completely removed by surgical planing to the level of the reticular dermis.(3) While dermabrasion can be used in the treatment of a wide variety of lesions, including actinic and seborrheic keratoses, angiofibromas, solar elastosis, and rhytides, it is particularly useful in the treatment of acne scars. (35) Although the advent of ablative and nonablative lasers has broadened the therapeutic armamentarium for skin resurfacing, the role of wire-brush surgery in the treatment of deep defects of the skin continues to be an important one. For the treatment of typical facial acne scars, in particular scars of the "boxcar" type, motorized dermabrasion is preferred over manual dermasanding. While microdermabrasion appears to at least transiently provide a mild improvement of acne-induced dyschromia and overall appearance, its impact on acne scarring is very limited compared to conventional dermabrasion. An understanding of the common clinical applications of dermabrasion, the advantages of the technique, and its limitations can improve outcomes and maximize patient satisfaction. The successful treatment of acne scarring can be difficult to achieve. Patients respond differently to treatments, and what works for one patient may not work for another. Often times, multiple techniques are required, and even then, only 50% to 75% improvement is seen in most patients.(11) Therefore, it is important to emphasize to the patient that acne scarring can be improved but never entirely reversed.(2) However, the treatment of patients with realistic expectations can be a mutually satisfying endeavor for both the healthcare provider and the patient.

REFERENCES

1. Kimball AB. Advances in the treatment of acne. J Reprod Med 2008; 53: 742–52.
2. Alam M, Dover JS. Treatment of acne scarring. Skin Therapy Lett 2006; 11: 7–9.
3. Harmon CB. Chapter 270: Dermabrasion. In: Fitzpatrick's Dermatology in General Medicine, 6th Edition. I.M. Freedberg AZE, K. Wolff, K. F. Austen, L.A. Goldsmith, S.I. Katz, ed. Vol. 2: McGraw-Hill Professional, 2003: 2536–7.
4. Campbell RM, Harmon CB. Dermabrasion in our practice. J Drugs Dermatol 2008; 7: 124–8.
5. Chapas AM, Brightman L, Sukal S et al. Successful treatment of acneiform scarring with CO2 ablative fractional resurfacing. Lasers Surg Med 2008; 40: 381–6.
6. Lawrence N, Mandy S, Yarborough J et al. History of dermabrasion. Dermatol Surg 2000; 26: 95–101.
7. Padilla RS & JM, Yarborough J. Chapter 28: Dermabrasion. In: Dermatologic Surgery. Ratz JL, ed. Philadelphia, PA: Lippincott-Raven Publishers, 1998: 473–84.
8. Kromayer E. Rotational instruments as a new tool in dermatologic surgery. Chir. Dermatol. Ztschr, 1905: 12: 26.

9. Kirsner RS. Wound healing. In: Dermatology. Bolognia JL, Jorizzo, Rapini, eds. 2nd edn. Mosby Elsevier, 2008: 2147–58.

10. Harmon CB, Zelickson BD, Roenigk RK et al. Dermabrasive scar revision. Immunohistochemical and ultrastructural evaluation. Dermatol Surg 1995; 21: 503–8.

11. Frith M, Harmon CB. Acne scarring: current treatment options. Dermatol Nurs 2006; 18: 139–42.

12. Goodman GJ, Baron JA. The management of postacne scarring. Dermatol Surg 2007; 33: 1175–88.

13. Jacob CI, Dover JS, Kaminer MS. Acne scarring: a classification system and review of treatment options. J Am Acad Dermatol 2001; 45: 109–17.

14. Alam M, Omura N, Kaminer MS. Subcision for acne scarring: technique and outcomes in 40 patients. Dermatol Surg 2005; 31: 310–7.

15. Rubenstein R, Roenigk HH Jr, Stegman SJ et al. Atypical keloids after dermabrasion of patients taking isotretinoin. J Am Acad Dermatol 1986; 15: 280–5.

16. Goodman G. Dermabrasion using tumescent anesthesia. J Dermatol Surg Oncol 1994; 20: 802–7.

17. Pinski JB. Dressings for dermabrasion: occlusive dressings and wound healing. Cutis 1986; 37: 471–6.

18. Spencer JM, Harmon CB. Chapter 36: Microdermabrasion and dermabrasion. In: Surgery of the Skin, Procedural Dermatology. J. Robinson CWH, R. Sengelmann, D. Siegel, ed. Mosby, 2005.

19. Alster T. Laser scar revision: comparison study of 585-nm pulsed dye laser with and without intralesional corticosteroids. Dermatol Surg 2003; 29: 25–9.

20. Grimes PE, Bhawan J, Kim J et al. Laser resurfacing-induced hypopigmentation: histologic alterations and repigmentation with topical photochemotherapy. Dermatol Surg 2001; 27: 515–20.

21. Monheit GD, Chastain MA. Chemical and Mechanical Skin Resurfacing. In: Dermatology. Bolognia JL, Jorizzo, Rapini, eds. 2nd edn. Mosby Elsevier, 2008: 2313–27.

22. Zisser M, Kaplan B, Moy RL. Surgical pearl: manual dermabrasion. J Am Acad Dermatol 1995; 33: 105–6.

23. Tsai RY, Wang CN, Chan HL. Aluminum oxide crystal microdermabrasion. A new technique for treating facial scarring. Dermatol Surg 1995; 21: 539–42.

24. Rivera AE. Acne scarring: a review and current treatment modalities. J Am Acad Dermatol 2008; 59: 659–76.

25. Spencer JM. Microdermabrasion. Am J Clin Dermatol 2005; 6: 89–92.

26. Freedman BM, Rueda-Pedraza E, Waddell SP. The epidermal and dermal changes associated with microdermabrasion. Dermatol Surg 2001; 27: 1031–3.

27. Karimipour DJ, Kang S, Johnson TM et al. Microdermabrasion: a molecular analysis following a single treatment. J Am Acad Dermatol 2005; 52: 215–23.

28. Rajan P, Grimes PE. Skin barrier changes induced by aluminum oxide and sodium chloride microdermabrasion. Dermatol Surg 2002; 28: 390–3.

29. Prausnitz MR, Langer R. Transdermal drug delivery. Nat Biotechnol 2008; 26: 1261–8.

30. Lee WR, Tsai RY, Fang CL et al. Microdermabrasion as a novel tool to enhance drug delivery via the skin: an animal study. Dermatol Surg 2006; 32: 1013–22.

31. Freedman BM. Hydradermabrasion: an innovative modality for nonablative facial rejuvenation. J Cosmet Dermatol 2008; 7: 275–80.

32. Freedman BM. Topical antioxidant application enhances the effects of facial microdermabrasion. J Dermatolog Treat 2008: 1–6.

33. Dermanetwork. Acne scarring. URL: www.dermanetwork.org/information/acne_scars.asp. In, 01/14/2009 (access date).

34. Savardekar P. Microdermabrasion. Indian J Dermatol Venereol Leprol 2007; 73: 277–9.

35. Roenigk HH Jr. Dermabrasion for miscellaneous cutaneous lesions (exclusive of scarring from acne). J Dermatol Surg Oncol 1977; 3: 322–8.

8 Fillers and fat transfer for treatment of acne scarring
Timothy Corcoran Flynn and Derek Jones

INTRODUCTION
Just as there is a high prevalence of acne vulgaris in the population, there is the resultant amount of scarring. A nice review by Rivera (1) discussed a study that looked at acne scarring in over 20,000 US citizens, in the age group of 1 through 74 years. (2) The prevalence of acne was found to be 68 per 1,000 people and acne scarring was found to be 1.7 per 1,000 people. Most adolescents have acne, occurring in 80% of girls and 90% of boys. Looking at people aged between 11 and 30 years, 80% have some amount of diagnosable acne. The study showed acne scarring to be present in 1.7 per 1,000 people. Another study of acne scarring evaluated 749 patients, all above 25 years of age. In this study, acne scarring was noted in 14% of the women and 11% of the men enrolled.

Acne scarring may be present in the population at an undesirable rate. It is known that of those suffering acne vulgaris, approximately 16% seek medical treatment and 74% wait greater than a year before seeking evaluation. Furthermore, the presence of acne among adolescents is often accepted as a "normal part of the teenage years." Because of the acceptance of this inflammatory condition, treatment may not be undertaken and acne scarring may result.

Acne scars can be understood as those scars that are a result of increased tissue proliferation, or, more commonly, scars that are the result of damage to tissue, causing tissue loss.(1) This chapter will deal with the use of filler substances to treat aspects of tissue loss as a result of acne.

ACNE SCARS AS A RESULT OF TISSUE LOSS
Scars amenable to treatment with filler substance or fat transfer are scars that are due to tissue loss. Jacob et al. (3) described classification of these atrophic scars as ice-pick, rolling, and boxcar scars. Ice-pick scars are small, deep voids of tissue, which can contain collagen links to the dermis or subcutaneous tissue. The scar openings are small and can be described as pits. These are commonly seen on the cheeks. Depressed or boxcar scars are described as shallow to deep, 1.5 to 4 mm in width. They have a sharply defined edge with steep, almost vertical placed walls. Soft, rolling scars can be seen on the face, which are >4 mm in diameter, having gently sloped edges that merge with the normal-appearing skin. There can be dermal or subdermal tethering, and subcision can be very helpful in treating these scars. Atrophic scars are an additional type of acne scar, in which widespread tissue damage results in a slightly wrinkled, soft texture overlying a depressed area. Occasionally underlying vasculature can be seen below it.

WHICH ACNE SCARS RESPOND BEST TO FILLERS AND FAT TRANSFER?
Just as there are a variety of methods to improve acne scarring, so there are a variety of ways in which fillers can be used in the treatment of acne scarring.

SUBCUTANEOUS VERSUS DERMAL FILLING
Fillers can be used in two basic ways for the improvement of atrophic or depressed acne scars. The first are fillers used in the skin to replace portions of the dermis that have been lost. The atrophic tissue or scar has created a depression in the skin. The goal of the filling is to elevate these scars and decrease the light-and-shadow play on the skin that makes these depressions visible. A variety of fillers can be used for this, but in general the authors favor collagen products. These are white-to-yellowish filler substances and may be placed more superficially than the hyaluronic acids in order to elevate the skin. They do not pose the risk of Tyndall effect that is found with some hyaluronic acids, imparting a blue hue to the skin. The second type of filling is general volume replacement (Figure 8.1). Many patients who have superficial or shallow atrophic scars observe an accentuation of these scars with age and the subsequent soft-tissue volume loss. Replacing the volume of the subcutaneous tissue through deeper fillers or autologous fat transplantation can stretch back out the skin and bring the skin to a more even tension and elevation. These techniques can also be used to minimize the accentuation of skin pores that is often seen with skin aging. The author favors calcium hydroxyapatite, fat transfer or poly-l-lactic acid as well as hyaluronic acids designed for deep use.

Many patients respond best with a combination of deep-volume replacement along with dermal filling. If filling is used in combination with resurfacing or punch elevation followed by resurfacing, improvement can be more significant.

It is important to not overpromise the degree of scar improvement possible through the use of filler substances. In general, in the authors practice, a 50% improvement is discussed with the patient. If a >50% improvement results, patients will be quite pleased.

TREATMENT OF ICE-PICK SCARS WITH FILLER SUBSTANCE
Filler substances are not the primary treatment of the ice-pick type scars. These are dermal fibrosis, causing a pit in the skin often found with a subcutaneous tether at the base of this thin scar. It is often times difficult to just fill the interior of the ice-pick scar. Instead, when filler substances are attempted the filler migrates into the surrounding normal tissues and as such, a

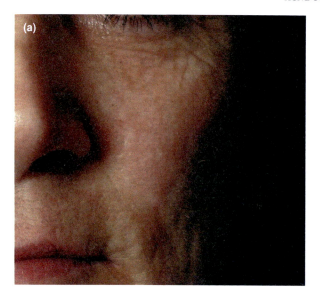 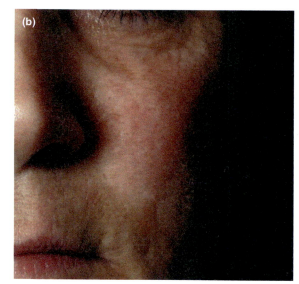

Figure 8.1 Effect of pure volume replacement on (A) aged, acne-scarred skin. Eight ml of normal saline was infiltrated into the prezygomatic cheek (B); volume replacement in itself can improve the appearance of acne-scarred skin.

"donut" of elevation occurs around the ice-pick type scar worsening the appearance. Many practitioners prefer the punch-excision or punch-elevation technique to the ice-pick scars, which is then followed by a CO_2 resurfacing or dermabrasion. However, there are select ice-pick type scars, which are not deep and which can benefit from filler substances. The author favors Cosmoderm® for this filling, as it is a very forgiving substance. In America we are looking forward to the use of EVOLENCE BREEZE®, a porcine collagen, which has shown promise. Again, care must be undertaken when filling the ice-pick-type scar.

ROLLING SCARS

Rolling scars are a result of dermal atrophy. Some of these scars can respond to filler treatments. Collagens and hyaluronic acids can be helpful for this purpose. When using hyaluronic acids one should select a hyaluronic acid with good cohesive flow and an ability to intercalate in between collagen bundles. It has been noted by Wang et al. (4), using Restylane® as the hyaluronic acid, that Restylane® placement within the dermis has been shown to increase type I collagen. It may be that repetitive uses of hyaluronic acids actually serve to build up a collagen layer within the skin.

BOXCAR-TYPE SCARS

Boxcar scars can respond to filler substances. However, their sharp edges and drop-off suggest the concomitant use of resurfacing techniques. Manual diamond fraise or wire-brush dermabrasion can be used to round off the edges of the scar prior to filler substance replacement, decreasing the shadow and "cliff-like effect." Filler substances can then be used at the base of the scar to elevate the center.

ATROPHIC SCARS

The practitioner who is attempting to improve atrophic scars must first determine whether these scars look worse because the atrophy of the skin has accentuated underlying vessels. If these vessels are present, causing a darker appearance to the scar, vascular lasers may be used to obliterate these vessels at the base of the scar. Once this achieved, replacement of the atrophic dermis with a filler substance may be very helpful. Collagen or hyaluronic acid may be used for this condition. Care must be taken to place these substances in the appropriate layer. Because of the atrophy of the skin it is possible, at times, to see the filler substances traveling too high within the dermis, creating small papules or visible tracts of filler substance. Practitioners should use care and time when filling the atrophic scars. Often times the atrophic scars are accompanied by underlying fat atrophy. Deeper filler substances such as poly-L-lactic acid or Radiesse® may be used to increase the volume in the deep subcutaneous soft tissue. This increase in volume will serve to stretch the skin and bring these atrophic scars up to a plane more even with the skin. Many patients have begun their scar treatment with filler substances targeted to the individual and scars and later progressed to procedures designed to replace deep-volume loss. Patients are often quite thrilled with the result and note that the dual treatment is helping them to achieve the appearance that they desire. This enthusiastic response demonstrates that patients and practitioners often focus on the individual scars, creating an uneven appearance to the skin and lack an appreciation of the concomitant volume loss with skin wrinkling, atrophy, and accentuation of the acne scars.

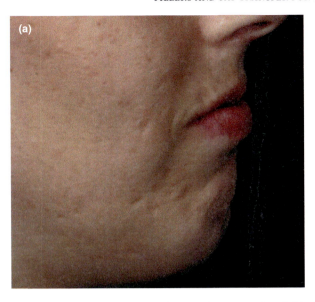 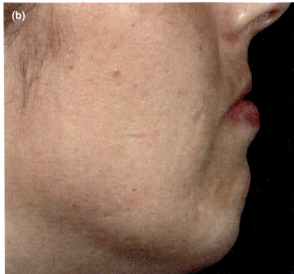

Figure 8.2 Patient with cheek and perioral acne scarring. (A) Before and (B) 2 weeks after treatment with injectable bovine collagen injected intradermally into the atrophic scars.

INDIVIDUAL FILLER SUBSTANCE USEFUL FOR TREATMENT OF ACNE SCARS

Collagens

Zyderm, Zyplast, Cosmoderm, Cosmoplast, Evolence, and Evolence Breeze are all collagens. However, they vary in their animal origins. The bovine-based products Zyderm and Zyplast have a long history, having been in use in the United States since 1977.(5) A team of investigators at Stanford University produced a stable implantable collagen and conducted a trial of human and bovine collagen in 28 patients, injecting the collagen into depressed acne scars, subcutaneous atrophy, wrinkling, and so on.(6) The contour defects were improved by 50% to 85%, and the early report showed maintenance from 3 to 18 months.

The Collagen Corporation was formed to produce Zyderm, the purified bovine collagen. This product was extensively studied, showing excellent results in acne scars. The original Zyderm I (35 mg/ml) was further concentrated, producing Zyderm II (65 mg/ml). Zyplast was developed by lightly cross linking collagen with gluteraldehyde. Zyplast is more resistant to protealytic degradation and less immunogenic.

These products continue to be useful in the appropriate patients (Figure 8.2). For fine acne scarring, Zyderm I is a very flexible and elegant product. It is injected in the skin at the appropriate intradermal level with the practitioner overcorrecting the acne scar to 150%. Zyderm II, the more concentrated product, can also be used but requires a bit more skill. Acne scars should be corrected to 100%. Certain patients may benefit from the thicker Zyplast product. Zyderm I and II are useful for shallow acne scars and excisional scars.(7) Any soft, superficial defect will be well served by Zyderm I and II. Deep acne scars can be treated with Zyplast and may also benefit from a Zyderm I or II overlay. It is important to remember that Zyderm I leaves 30% of the volume injected when it condenses on implantation. Zyderm II leaves approximately 60% of the injected material behind.

Because these products are bovine in nature, it is important to take a history of an anaphylactoid event or previous sensitivity to bovine collagen. Patients desiring Zyderm or Zyplast should undergo a skin test. The skin-test syringe contains 0.3 ml of Zyderm I. It is usually placed in the volar forearm. The site is evaluated by the patient at 48 to 72 hours and again at 4 weeks. A positive skin test is indurated, tender, and has redness that persists 6 hours or longer after implantation. A positive skin test response will be seen in approximately 3% of people, and most of the reactions will become manifest within 72 hours. We recommend a second test as an additional precaution. The product contains lidocaine, so beware of a patient's lidocaine allergy.

Cosmoderm and Cosmoplast are dermal fillers prepared from human fibroblasts grown under controlled conditions.(8) Clinical studies have indicated very little tissue reactivity and so no skin test is required for these. These products have been approved by the Food and Drug Administration in 2003. These products contain 0.3% lidocaine. While the products are excellent for use in acne scarring, many practitioners have reported that the longevity of these products is less than with the bovine preparations. Nonetheless, these products are well tolerated by patients and well-liked particularly by those patients with fine acne scarring in the cheeks (Figure 8.3).

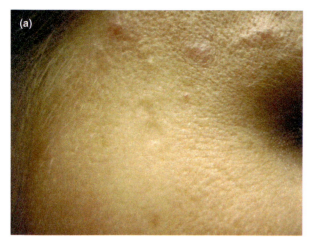

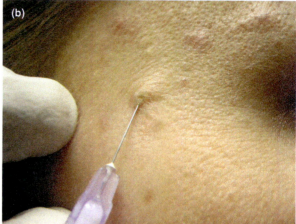

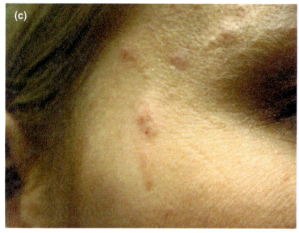

Figure 8.3 (A) Before, (B) during, and (C) immediately after varicella scar is filled with CosmoDerm collagen. Note intradermal implantation with yellowish discoloration as the material flows into the dermis. Overcorrection of scars is recommended with this product.

Cross-linked porcine collagen is sold under the name of Evolence and Evolence Breeze.(9) Natural porcine collagen is digested with pepsin to create a monumeric collagen and then the immunogenic telopeptides are removed. This produces a nonimmunogenic polymerized collagen. No skin testing is required. The company reports the use of a novel matrix of cross-linking, which gives a longevity of up to 1 year. Evolence has a role in treating acne scarring, but it is a thick product. It should be massaged when placed into the tissue and may have a tendency to form lumps when used for acne scarring. Its sister product, Evolence Breeze, has a better role for treatment of acne scars. This product is available in Europe, but is not yet available for use in the United States.

Hyaluronic Acids

Hyaluronic acids are a natural filler substance particularly suited for treatment of aging skin. Hyaluronic acid is a major component of the extracellular matrix, a polysaccharide with a high turnover rate.(10) Its function in the skin is in part to bind and retain water. However, as a person ages the amount of

HA in the skin is reduced, which decreases the volume of the skin, leading to drooping and visible wrinkles. Repeated sun exposure decreases the amount of HA in the dermis. By replacing HA in the skin, the youthful appearance can be restored, replacing the lost HA and binding the water.

Hyaluronic acid fillers can be used in the treatment of acne scars. One caveat is that these fillers, if placed too high in the dermis, may exhibit a slight blue tint. This has been particularly noted with the Restylane family of products. Hyaluronic acids are thus suitable for deeper filling. They can be used in the mid-dermis to the subcutaneous dermis with some large particle-type hyaluronic acids placed deep within the tissue to revolumize the underlying soft tissue and distend the acne scars.

There are a variety of injectable hyaluronic acid products available. They can be differentiated by (a) molecular weight, (b) concentration, (c) method and degree of cross-linking, (d) particle versus monophasic technology, (5) avian versus bacterial origin.

Most hyaluronic acid manufacturers are now seeking approval to allow the FDA to sell them mixed with an anesthetic such as lidocaine. However, most practitioners mix a small amount of lidocaine in with the hyaluronic acids by the use of a female-to-female Luer-Lok injector. This greatly reduces the discomfort of the hyaluronic acid injection.

Hyaluronic acids are an excellent filler in that they are long lasting, naturally appearing, smooth to the touch, rarely allergenic, and can be reversed with the use of hyaluronidase. For intradermal filling the use of Restylane and Juvederm Ultra can be used in those scars that have a dermal atrophic appearance. However, these products must be placed in the lower portion of the dermis in order to "lift" the normal-appearing dermis up to the level of the skin. The monophasic technology of the Juvederm family of products is much preferable in that it tends to integrate this product better into the dermal collagen; the particle products such as Hylaform, Captique, or Restylane and Perlane may tend to agglutinate within the scar (data awaiting publication).

Mid-face volumizing with hyaluronic acids can be helpful in a patient with acne scarring that has an accentuation due to volume loss.(11, 12) Products such as Restylane, SubQ, or Voluma have a greater "lift" capacity. The Restylane SubQ product has the same properties as Restylane products, except that the gel particle sizes are larger compared to Perlane. Voluma, within the Juvederm family of products, is a monophasic, 20-mg/ml hyaluronic acid product with a lower molecular weight and a higher cross-linking ratio, which allows for retention of structure after deep injection. These products are used very similarly to autologous fat in that the volume replacement can reduce the appearance of the atrophic acne scars.

Hyaluronic acids also have the advantage of being reversible. Hyaluronidase can be used to melt implanted hyaluronic acid. This is commonly done if pooling, ridging, or nodules occur.(13)

Poly-L-Lactic Acid

Poly-l-lactic acid is a biodegradable, synthetic polymer, molecularly similar to the vicryl suture.(14) The product is known as Sculptra in the United States, which comes as a sterile, freeze-dried powder. The powder is reconstituted into a suspension 24 hours prior to injection. When injected into the subcutaneous tissue poly-l-lactic acid causes immediate and delayed volume restoration. The material, when injected, immediately causes edema, but gradually fibroblast proliferation and neocollagenesis is formed. Sculptra has its main benefit as a deep-volume replacer and thus may improve lax skin that contains atrophic acne scars. It is very important to place this product deeply through multiple injections. We frequently use a cross-hatch linear retrograde injection technique in order to increase volume of the deep tissues. It is important to note that there have been several reports of papule and nodule development, and these have been related to either intradermal injection or placement under thin skin, such as the periocular area.(15) This product is designed to be used in multiple treatment sections approximately 1 to 2 months apart. Depending on the degree of revolumization, anywhere from 2 to 6 vials of Sculptra may be needed.

Sculptra has been directly shown to benefit acne scars directly in a report by Beer.(16) Poly-l-lactic acid was injected serially at or near the sites of the acne scars. The investigator reported significant reduction in acne scar size and severity. Subjects also noted a gradual improvement. Sadove (17) also reported success in atrophic acne scarring using Sculptra in two patients.

Calcium hydroxyapatite

Calcium hydroxyapatite is a naturally occurring substance used for over a decade in reconstructive surgery.(18) Radiesse is a semipermanent biodegradable soft-tissue filler composed of calcium hydroxyapatite microspheres in a gel carrier. This product is useful as a deep-volume filler that also builds new collagen. It is helpful in acne scars by building up new subdermal collagen underlying loose skin with acne scars. The product is placed deeply, in the immediate subcutaneous plane or deeper, and the gel carrier is gradually phagocytized, leaving the calcium hydroxyapatite microspheres behind. This acts as a scaffold that allows fibroblasts to attach to the scaffold and lay down a collageneous extracellular matrix that becomes integrated into the tissues and adds volume (Figure 8.4). The microspheres are gradually metabolized over a period of 9 to 18 months. It does not cause ossification and is radio opaque; however, it does not interfere with x-ray or CT-scan interpretation.(19)

Radiesse is a robust filler with good lift capacity.(20, 21) It can be mixed by the practitioner with 2% lidocaine prior to injection to minimize the pain of injection. The syringe comes with 1.3 cc of product, and an excellent 27G 1.25-inch needle. A linear retrograde injection technique should be employed into deep tissues or the subdermal plane. A slow injection technique with small aliquot deposition may help the appearance of atrophic acne scarred skin. It is not recommended to be used as a dermal filler. Radiesse can be a wonderful initial volumizing filler, with collagen or hyaluronic acids used on top of the Radiesse.

FAT TRANSPLANTATION

Fat transplantation (22, 23), or the idea of moving fat from one portion of the body to another, has a more than 100 years history. Modern techniques of fat transplantation have roots back to 1976 when the idea of suctioning fat was developed by the Fishers. The excellent pharmacologic work of Dr. Jeff Kline led to the modern tumescent liposuction technique, which provides physicians with an almost endless supply of viable adipose tissue. Using tumescent anesthesia, fat can be readily harvested and transferred to a syringe for reimplantation. Fat transfer can be helpful in acne scarring by restoring the loss of subcutaneous fat and replacing volume, which stretches the overlying skin and distends the acne scars. Patients who are particularly good candidates for fat transplantation include the acne-scarred patient who has a thin, atrophic face. Many of these older patients can benefit from a pan-facial lipoaugmentation concurrent with the specific injections designed to minimize the acne scarring.

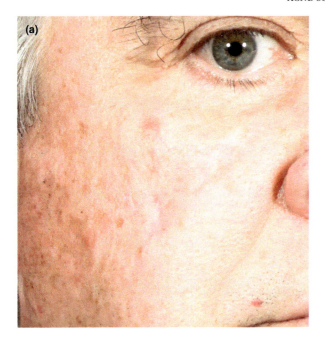
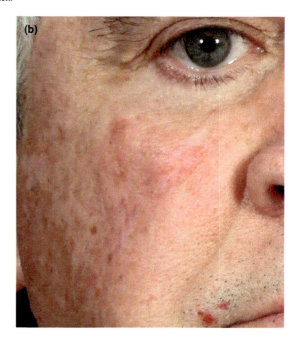

Figure 8.4 (A) Before and (B) after of a surgical scar on acne-scarred skin. Calcium hydroxyapatite was used deeply, and, after 6 weeks, was superficially overlaid with Cosmoderm injectable collagen.

Donor fat is extracted from a donor site with common areas being the thigh, buttocks, or inner knee.(24) Tumescent anesthesia is used with a harvesting cannula; most commonly a 3-mm, open, cobra-tipped cannula with a Luer-Lok is used to harvest the fat into a 10 ml syringe. Gentle aspiration is essential to not disrupt the adipocytes. Many practitioners centrifuge the fat prior to transferring it into 1-cc Luer-Lok syringes.

The fat can then be placed deeply into the patient's facial skin that underlies the atrophic acne areas. It is helpful to use local anesthesia, a No-Kor needle, and a blunt-tipped 18-gauge fat infiltrator. The goal is to place multiple tiny deposits of harvested "fat cylinders" within several deep planes of the cheeks. We tell our patients that they should expect approximately 3 to 4 treatment sessions before we achieve an ideal result. It is also possible to freeze the fat (25), allowing for only one harvesting session followed by the 3 to 4 fat transplantation sessions. Fat transplantation is not to be used as an intradermal implant.

LIQUID INJECTABLE SILICONE

Liquid injectable silicone (LIS) is composed of polydimethylsiloxane. Approved by the FDA as an injectable retinal tamponade for retinal detachment, LIS comes in two forms: Silikon®-1000 (Alcon Laboratories; Fort Worth, TX) and AdatoSil® 5000 (Bausch and Lomb). The viscosity of silicone, which is reflected in the number at the end of the brand name, is expressed in centistokes (cS) units, with 100 cS being the viscosity of water and increasing values reflecting more viscous products. Although it is not FDA approved for injectable soft-tissue augmentation,

Silikon®-1000 is commonly used legally off-label for this purpose, considering its lower viscosity and ability to be injected through smaller gauge needles, (26)

Liquid silicone was first used as an injectable filler in the 1950s. It became more widely used in the 1970s and 1980s, although there was no standardized FDA-approved product and many "medical-grade" silicone oils of varying purity were injected often in large bolus form, leading to frequent product migration and foreign-body inflammatory reactions. In the 1980s, mounting cases of adverse events led health authorities to investigate the cosmetic safety of this product. Several reports of ulceration, connective tissue disease, granulomas, and filler migration led to the legal banning of LIS for cosmetic indications in the early 1990s. In the late 1990s, two important FDA provisions let LIS emerge on the market again after a brief hiatus. First, Silikon®-1000 and AdatoSil®-5000 were FDA approved for treating retinal detachment. A second concurrent event, the passage of the FDA Modernization Act, made it legal for FDA-approved injectable devices to be used off-label for other indications as long as such provisions were not openly advertised and physicians based their decision to use the device off-label on unique, individual patient needs.

Currently, opinion on liquid injectable silicone is polarized between opponents and advocates. Opponents advocate that despite use of proper technique and products, serious adverse events are common and unpredictable. Advocates rely on a wealth of anecdotal data to argue that liquid injectable silicone is safe and effective as long as three rules are employed: (1) Use

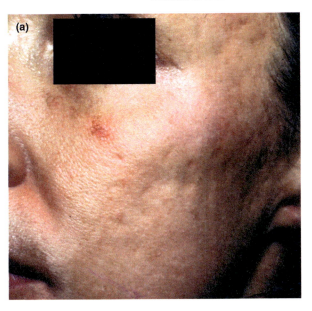
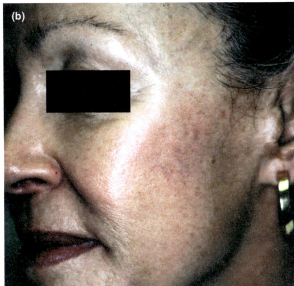

Figure 8.5 (A) Pretreatment acne scarring. (B) Thirty years postinjection of 1.8 ccs of LIS, injected in six treatments over four years. Reproduced with permission from Barnett JG et al.(27)

highly purified FDA approved LIS; (2) employ microdroplet serial-puncture technique, defined as multiple injection of 0.01 cc into the subdermal plane or deeper at 3 to 5 mm intervals with no second pass; and (3) use small volumes (0.5 ccs for smaller defects and up to 2 ccs for larger areas of atrophy) at each session with multiple sessions staged at monthly intervals or longer. Gradual fibroplasia ensues around each silicone microdroplet anchoring it in place and contributing to the ultimate result.

Liquid injectable silicone is useful as both an immediate and long-lasting treatment for broad-based, depressed acne scars and is the only filler substance that maintains precision and permanence in improving and/or correcting these types of acne scar defects. A recent report describes five patients with a history of acne scarring who showed improvements from injections of liquid silicone at the initial treatment session and lasting over a 10-, 15-, and 30-year follow-up period (Figure 8.5).(27) Monthly liquid-silicone injections were employed using the microdroplet, multiple-injection approach. Results describe the safety, effectiveness, and precision of silicone in addition to highlighting the fact that its permanence is what distinguishes it from other filler materials. It was concluded that liquid injectable silicone is a precise and permanent filling substance used for soft-tissue augmentation and can improve and/or eliminate depressed, broad-based acne scars with the microdroplet, multiple-injection approach.

Furthermore, in a recent testimony, 35 skin biopsies obtained from target areas where LIS had been previously injected for correction of depressed facial scars were examined by light microscopy.(28) The investigators found that LIS remained in

the target areas in 100% of the cases biopsied without inducing any significant adverse complications. In several of the cases, LIS had been injected many years (up to 23 years) before the tissue was biopsied. However, for the unique and disfiguring defects associated with serious acne scarring, patients and physicians should be aware of this excellent treatment modality that most frequently produces cosmetically superior and more durable results than currently available less permanent options

REFERENCES

1. Rivera AE. Acne scarring: a review of current treatment modalities. J Am Acad Dermatol 2008; 59: 659–76.
2. Johnson MR, Roberts J. Skin conditions and related need for medical care among persons 1–74 Years, United States, 1971–1974. Washington DC: US Department of Health, Education and Welfare, Vital Health Statistics, Series II, No 212, Nov 1978.
3. Jacobs I, Dover JS, Kamien MS. Acne scarring: a classification system and review of treatment options. J Am Acad Dermatol 2004; 22: 434–8.
4. Wang F, Garza LA, Kang S et al. In vivo stimulation of De Novo collagen production caused by cross-linked hyaluronic acid dermal filler injection in photodamaged human skin. Arch Dermatol 2007; 143: 155–63.
5. Klein AW. Skin filling: collagen and other injectables of the skin. Dermatol Clin 2001; 19: 491–508.
6. Knapp TR, Kaplan EM, Daniels JR. Injectable collagen for soft tissue augmentation. Plastic Reconstr Surgery 1977; 60: 389.

7. Bailin MD, Bailin PM. Case Studies: correction of surgical scars, acne scars and rhytids with Zyderm and Zyplast implants. J Dermatol Surg Oncol 1988; (Supp 1): 31.

8. Bauman L. Cosmoderm/Cosmoplast (human bioengineered collagen) for the aging face. Facial Plast Surg 2004; 20: 125–8.

9. Beer K. Evolence: the thing of shapes to come. Skin Aging 2007; 15: 22–3.

10. Tezel A, Fredrickson GH. The science of hyaluronic acid sub-dermal fillers. J Cosmet Laser Ther 2008; 10(1): 35–42.

11. Raspaldo H. Volumizing effect of a new hyaluronic acid sub-dermal filler: a retrospective analysis based on 102 cases. J Cosmet Laser Ther 2008; 10(3): 134–42.

12. Lowe NJ, Grover R. Injectable hyaluronic acid implant for malar and mental enhancement. Dermatol Surg 2006; 32(7): 881–5.

13. Brody HJ. Use of hyaluronidase in the treatment of granulomatous hyaluronic acid reactions or unwanted hyaluronic acid misplacement. Dermat Surg 2005: 31: 893–7.

14. Lacombe V. Sculptra: a stimulatory filler. Facial Plast Surg 2009; 25: 95–9.

15. Stewart DB, Morganroth GS, Mooney MA et al. Management of visible granulomas following periorbital injection of poly-L-lactic acid. Ophthal Plast Reconstr Surg 2007; 23(4): 298–301.

16. Beer K. A single-center, open-label study on the use of poly-L-lactic acid for the treatment of moderate to severe scarring from acne on varicella. Dermatol Surg 2007; 33: 5159–67.

17. Sadove R. Injectable poly-l-lactic: a novel sculpting agent for the treatment of dermal fat atrophy after severe acne. Aesthetic Plast Surg 2009; 33: 113–6.

18. Goldberg D. Calcium hydroxylapatite. In: Fillers in cosmetic dermatology. Abingdon, England: Informa UK Ltd; 2006.

19. Carruthers A, Liebeskind M, Carruthers J, Forster BB. Radiographic and computed tomographic studies of calcium hydroxylapatite for treatment of HIV-associated facial lipoatrophy and correction of nasolabial folds. Dermatol Surg 2008; 34(Supp 1): S78–84.

20. Smith S, Busso M, McClaren M, Bass LS. A randomized, bilateral, prospective comparison of calcium hydroxylapatite microspheres versus human-based collagen for the correction of nasolabial folds. Dermatol Surg 2007; 33(Supp 2): S112–21.

21. Sadick NS, Katz BE, Roy DA. Multicenter, 47-month study of safety and efficacy of calcium hydroxylapatite for soft tissue augmentation of nasolabial folds and other areasw of the face. Dermatol Surg 2007; 33(Supp 2): S122–6.

22. Donofrio L. Structural Lipoaugmentation in narins R.S. Cosmetic Surgery, Marcel Dekker New York, 2001.

23. Fournier PF. Facial recontouring with fat grafting. Dermatol Clin 1990; 8: 523–37.

24. Kaufman MR, Bradley JP, Dickinson B et al. Autologous fat transfer national consensus survey: trends in techniques for harvesting, preparation, application and perception of short and long term results. Plast Reconst Surg 2007; 119: 322–31.

25. Jackson RF, Frozen fat: Does it work? Am J Cosmet Surg 1997; 14: 339–43.

26. Jones DH, Carruthers A, Orentreich D et al. Highly purified 1000-cSt silicone oil for treatment of human immunodeficiency, virus-associated facial lipoatrophy: an open pilot trial. Dermatol Surg 2004; 30(10): 1279–86.

27. Barnett JG, Barnett CR. Treatment of acne scars with liquid silicone injections: 30-year perspective. Dermatol Surg 2005; 31: 1542–9.

28. Zappi E, Barnett JG, Zappi M, Barnett CR. The long-term host response to liquid silicone injected during soft tissue augmentation procedures: a microscopic appraisal. Dermatol Surg 2007; 33(Supp 2): 5186–92.

9 Needling
Gabriella Fabbrocini, Nunzio Fardella, and Ambra Monfrecola

KEY FEATURE

- Innovative and useful technique for acne scars treatment as an alternative to laser, chemical peelings, and dermabrasion.
- Induction of new dermal collagen synthesis and deposition by activation of a local inflammatory response.
- The skin is not damaged. The epidermis and particularly the stratum corneum remain intact.
- There are no risks of hyperpigmentation.
- The healing phase is short and the treatment can be repeated.

INTRODUCTION

Skin needling, percutanous collagen induction (PCI), collagen induction therapy (CIT), dry tattooing, needle dermabrasion, intradermabrasion, dermal remodeling, multirepannic collagen actuation, intradermabrasion (MCA), these are all names for the same treatment.

Skin needling is a procedure that involves using a sterile roller comprised of a series of fine, sharp needles to puncture the skin. Performed under local anaesthetic with sedation, the device is "rolled" over the surface affected by acne scars to create many microscopic channels deep into the dermis of the skin, which stimulates your own body to produce new collagen.

HISTORY

Skin needling has been performed for many years, using a variety of instruments, to soften depressed scars and deep lines. Dr Philippe Simonin, a Swiss-French dermatologist, published his results in *Baran's Cosmetic Dermatology* in 1994, but his ground-breaking technique, which he named electroridopuncture (ERP), remained largely unknown to the wider medical community. In 1995 Orentreich and Orentreich (1) described "subcision" as a way of building up connective tissue beneath retracted scars and wrinkles. Desmond Fernandes (2), simultaneously and independently, used a similar technique to treat the upper lip by inserting a 15-gauge needle into the skin and then tunneling under the wrinkles in various directions, parallel to the skin surface. Dr. Andre Camirand, a plastic surgeon, had an important publication in 1997, describing his experience with this method. On a number of his patients with facial hypochromic scars, he tattooed the scars with a skin-color pigment. After 1 to 2 years, they noticed that even though the pigment was long gone, it was replaced by actual melanin, while the scars were immensely improved in texture, appearance, and color. This gave the idea that trepanation (coming from the Greek word Trepanon: to bore) of scars with the tattoo gun was responsible for the improvement and the repigmentation of the scar. They

came up with the idea that puncturing of the scar with a tattoo gun alone, without pigment, would in a way break down the scar collagen, cause realignment, and stimulate melanogenesis. The results of repetitive sessions on scars were reported by Camirand to be much better and typically consistent, as all of his patients profited aesthetically from this type of treatment. Although this technique can be used on extensive areas, it was laboriously slow, and the holes in the epidermis were too close and too shallow.

All these techniques worked because the needles break old collagen strands in the most superficial layer of the dermis that tether scars or wrinkles. It is presumed that this process promotes removal of damaged collagen and induces more collagen immediately under the epidermis. Dr. Fernandes believed that the standard technique of tattooing was too superficial to give good effects for thicker scars or for stimulating collagenosis in the reticular dermis. Needles need to penetrate relatively deeply to stimulate the production of elastin fibers oriented from the deep layers of the dermis to the surface. Based on these principles, Desmond Fernandes designed a special tool for PCI, consisting of a rolling barrel with microneedles at regular intervals; in 1999 he presented his findings on needling at a conference in San Francisco. This presentation was instrumental in getting the information out to the medical community.

PATHOPHYSIOLOGY

PCI results from the natural response to wounding of the skin, even though the wound is minute and mainly subcutaneous. When a needle penetrates into the skin, it causes some localized damage and bleeding by rupturing fine blood vessels. A completely different picture emerges when thousands of fine pricks are placed close to each other. This promotes the normal wound healing that develops in **three phases** (Figure 9.1). The inflammation (**Phase 1**) starts soon after the injury: Platelets are important in causing clotting and releasing chemotactic factors, which cause an invasion of other platelets, leucocytes, and fibroblasts. After the platelets have been activated by exposure to thrombin and collagen, they release numerous cytokines. This process involves a complex concatenation of numerous factors that are important in

1. controlling the formation of a clot (e.g., fibrinogen, fibronectin, von Willebrand factor, thrombospondin, ADP, and thromboxane);
2. increasing vascular permeability, which then allows the neutrophils to pass through the vessel walls and enter the damaged area;
3. attracting neutrophils and monocytes;
4. recruiting fibroblasts into the wounded area. Of special interest in understanding the action of Skin Needling are FGF, PDGF, TGF-a, TGF-b, connective tissue activating peptide III, and neutrophil activating peptide 2.

ABLATIVE TECHNIQUES vs. DERMAROLLER

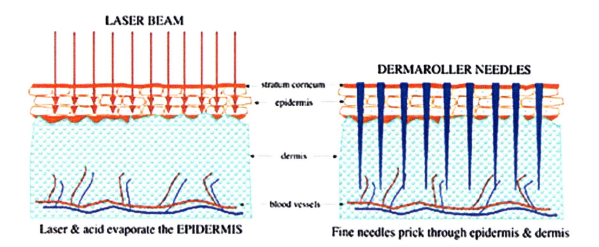

LASER BEAM

DERMAROLLER NEEDLES

stratum corneum

epidermis

dermis

blood vessels

Laser & acid evaporate the EPIDERMIS

Fine needles prick through epidermis & dermis

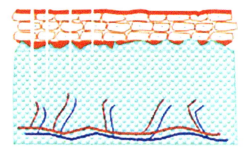

evaporated epidermis

A 2nd degree burn wound is set.
Inflammation, profilaration and maturation
can take month.

Pricking channels close within 1 hour.
Skin and epidermis stay intact.
Healing process starts immediately!

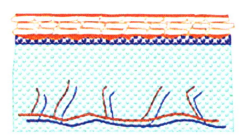

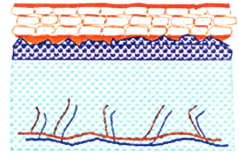

A new, relatively thin collagen layer grows.
The skin in total becomes thinner. A second
treatment in general is not possible.

A new and additional collagen layer is set
close to the corium. The skin becomes thicker.
Treatment can be repeated many times.

Figure 9.1 Ablative Techniques vs. Derma Roller (from www.dermaroller.de, with permission).

As time passes, probably about 5 days in the case of skin needling, (**Phase 2**) neutrophils are replaced by monocytes. The monocytes differentiate into macrophages and phagocytose the decaying neutrophils. They remove cellular debris and release several growth factors including platelet-derived growth factor, fibroblast growth factor, TGF-b, and TGF-a, which stimulate the migration and proliferation of fibroblasts and the production and modulation of extracellular matrix. Keratinocytes, the main cells in this case, change in morphology and become mobile to cover the gap in the basement membrane. When the keratinocytes have joined together, they start producing all the components to reestablish the basement membrane with laminin and collagen types IV and VII. A day or two after PCI, the keratinocytes start proliferating and act more in thickening the epidermis than in closing the defect. Initially after PCI, the disruption of blood vessels causes a moderate amount of hypoxia. The low-oxygen tension stimulates the fibroblast to produce more TGF-b, platelet-derived growth factor (PDGF) and endothelial growth factor (EGF). Procollagen MRNA is also upregulated, but this cannot cause collagen formation because oxygen is required, which occurs only when revascularization occurs. Prevascularization occurs quite soon after needling. TGF- is a powerful chemotoxic agent for fibroblasts that migrate into the wound at about 48 hours after injury and starts producing collagen I and III, elastin, glycosaminoglycans, and proteoglycans. Collagen type III is the dominant form of collagen in the early wound-healing phase and becomes maximal 5 to 7 days after injury. The collagen is laid down in the upper dermis just below the basal layer of the epidermis. Although the injury in skin needling extends deeper than the adnexal structures, because the epithelial wounds are simply cleft, myofibroblast wound contraction may not play a part in the healing. A number of proteins and enzymes are important for fibroplasia and angiogenesis that develop at the same time. Anoxia, TGF-b, and fibroblast growth factor and other growth factors play an important part in angiogenesis. Fibroblasts release insulin-like growth factor that is an important stimulant for proliferation of fibroblasts themselves and endothelial cells. Insulin-like growth factor is essential in neovascularisation. Insulin-like growth factor or somatomedin-C also is one of the main active agents for growth hormone. Integrins facilitate the interaction of the fibroblasts, endothelial cells, and keratinocytes.

Tissue remodeling (**Phase 3**) continues for months after the injury and is mainly done by the fibroblasts. By the fifth day after injury, the fibronectin matrix is laid down along the axis in which fibroblasts are aligned and in which collagen will be laid down. TGF-b and other growth factors play an important part in the formation of this matrix. Collagen type III is laid down in the upper dermis just below the basal layer of the epidermis and is gradually replaced by collagen type I over a period of a year or more, which gives increased tensile strength. The matrix metalloproteinases (MMPs) are essential for the conversion process.(2)

Recently, a new hypothesis has been proposed to explain the PCI mechanism of action (3): When CIT (collagen induction therapy) is performed correctly using a high-quality device, the fine microneedles that penetrate the skin do so only superficially. The formation of new tissue (wound healing: inflammation-proliferation-maturation) is a complex series of reactions and interactions among cells and mediators. But it seems that these processes are somewhat cut short, when the skin is treated with needles. As a series of needles—not longer than 1.5 mm—do not set a wound in the classical sense; according to this theory, bioelectricity—also called demarcation current—triggers the cascade of growth factors immediately to the maturation phase. When stainless steel microneedles penetrate the skin they set fine wounds. Cells react to this intrusion with a "demarcation current" (Figure 9.2–9.3). This demarcation current is additionally increased by the needles own electrical potential. In some very interesting findings, the membrane of a living cell has been shown to have a resting electrical potential of -70 mV. The interior of the cell is charged negatively in contrast to the positive external surface. The electrical potential depends highly on the transport mechanisms. If a single acupuncture needle come close to a cell, the inner electrical potential quickly rises to -100 mV and more. The electrical potential difference is typical in the wound-healing process. The materials that penetrate the membrane are ionic and cells change the membrane potential by losing or gaining ions. Relative to its size, the cell membrane potential is enormous. On average, its thickness is 70 to 100 nm. This would be equivalent to a 10-million-volt potential difference over 1 meter. It can be further hypothesized that microneedles do not cause overt injury in the classical sense. The body is only somehow 'fooled' into believing that an injury has occurred! Cell membranes react to the local change in electrical potential with increased cell activity and with the release of potassium ion, proteins, and growth factors.

TECHNOLOGY

- **Indications**
    - Acne scarring: By treating acne rolling scars (Grade 2–3) with skin needling, the skin becomes thicker, and the results are superior to dermabrasion.
    - Scars, if they are white, they can become more skin colored.
    - To restore skin tightness in the early stages of facial aging.
    - Stretch marks.
    - Fine wrinkles.
    - Lax skin on the arms and abdomen.
- **Controindications**
    - Patients who have not pretreated their skin with vitamin A or alpha Hydroxi-Acids.
    - Presence of skin cancers, warts, solar keratoses, or any skin infection. The needles may disseminate abnormal cells by implantation.
    - Active acne or herpes labialis infections in the face or impetigo lesions anywhere on the body.
    - For patients on any anticoagulant therapy like warfarin, heparin, and other oral anticoagulants, the presence of these drugs may cause excessive, uncontrolled bleeding. Patients previously on such treatment should have their coagulation status checked before the treatment

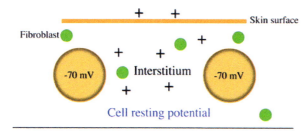

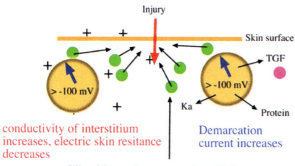

Figure 9.2 Cell resting potential before and after an injury (from www.dermaroller.de, with permission).

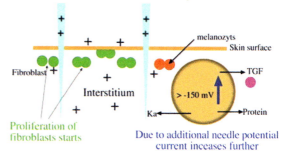

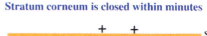

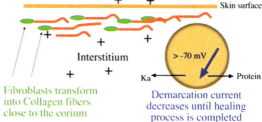

Figure 9.3 Activation of "Demarcation Currents" induced by stainless steel micro-needles induces fibroblasts' proliferation followed by synthesis of new collagen in the upper dermis (from www.dermaroller.de, with permission).

to confirm that they have a normal clotting/bleeding profile.

- For patients who take aspirin daily for medical or health reasons, the medication should be stopped at least 3 days before the procedure.
- Patients allergic to local anesthetic agents or general anesthesia should be assessed by a specialist anesthetist before treatment.
- Patients on chemotherapy, high doses of corticosteroids, or radiotherapy.
- Patients with uncontrolled diabetes mellitus.
- Patients who had facial surgery in the past 6 months.
- Patients with scars that are less than 6 months old.
- Patients who had "permanent" fillers, injected in the past 6 months.
- Patients with an extremely rare but severe form of keloid scarring in which virtually every pinprick becomes a keloid. Patients often have keloids on the palms of the hands or soles of the feet.

• Advantages
- Skin needling does not damage the skin. Histology has shown that the skin is indistinguishable from normal skin and that the epidermis may show more dermal papillae.
- Skin becomes thicker, with a great increase in collagen deposition and significantly more elastin.
- The healing phase is short and within 5 days the patients can go out in public.

- Topical numbing agents can be used to make the procedure comfortable. Very little discomfort posttreatment.
- Skin Needling can be safely performed on all skin colours and types. There is no risk of postinflammatory hyperpigmentation (pigmentation of the skin as a result of skin trauma) as the melanocytes remain, like the dermis, intact during skin needling. This is the major distinguishing safety feature when comparing skin needling and other invasive procedures that are used to treat deep lines and depressed scars, that is, laser resurfacing, deep chemical peels, and dermabrasion.
- There is reduced risk of infection.
- May be safely done in people with darker pigmented skin, without fear of hyperpigmentation.
- Sun sensitivity is a major and enduring problem in laser resurfacing, whereas after needling of the skin, the horny layer rapidly returns to its original thickness, and the skin is no longer sun sensitive.
- It is not as expensive as laser resurfacing.
- A major advantage is that needling can be performed on people who have had laser resurfacing or have thin skin.
- If the result after needling is not satisfactory, it can be repeated without any risk.
- A change can occur in dilated blood vessels that may disappear. Telangiectasia generally improves because

the vessels are ruptured in so many places that they cannot be repaired.

- **Disadvantages**
  - This procedure is relatively bloody, much the same as dermabrasion.
  - Skin needling cannot achieve as intense a deposition of collagen as laser resurfacing, but the treatment can be repeated to get even better results that will last as long, if not longer, as laser resurfacing.
- **Combination Possibilities**
  - Skin needling is a procedure that ensures better results if it's associated to alpha hydroxyacids treatment. Furthermore, as it has been shown that it promotes the transdermal penetration of drugs; this procedure can be used to improve the penetration of sebostatic agents in order to prevent the appearance of acne lesions that can develop into scars.

TECHNICAL PROCEDURES

Patient Preparation

The first step toward skin health is to topically replace photo-sensitive vitamin A and the other antioxidants, vitamins C and E and carotenoids, which are normally lost on exposure to light. Vitamin A is utterly essential for the normal physiology of skin and yet it is destroyed by exposure to light so that it is prevented from exerting its important influence on skin and preserving collagen. Vitamin A in physiologic doses will stimulate cell growth, the release of growth factors, angiogenesis, and the production of healthy new collagen. The DNA effects of vitamin A interact in parallel with the growth factors released by PCI. Adequate nourishment of the skin with vitamin A will ensure that the metabolic processes for collagen production will be maximized and the skin will heal as rapidly as possible. Vitamin C is similarly important for collagen formation but is destroyed by exposure to blue light. Both of these vitamins need to be replaced every day so that the natural protection and repair of DNA can be maintained. As a result, the skin will take on a more youthful appearance.

The skin is routinely prepared by using topical vitamin A and C and antioxidants for at least 3 weeks, but preferably for 3 months if the skin is very sun damaged. It can be used also a topical product containing alpha-omega HA, omega-hydroxyacides, enoxolone, and zinc. If the stratum corneum is thickened and rough, a series of mild TCA peels (2.5%–5% TCA) will get the surface of the skin prepared for needling and maximize the result.

At first, facial skin must be disinfected, then a topical anesthetic (EMLA) is applied leaving for 60 minutes (Figure 9.4). The skin-needling procedure is realized by rolling a performed tool on the skin areas affected by acne scars.

Actually there is a number of skin rollers available for professional and home use that come in many different needle lengths, diameters and numbers, which can make it very confusing for their users. In an attempt to determine the best

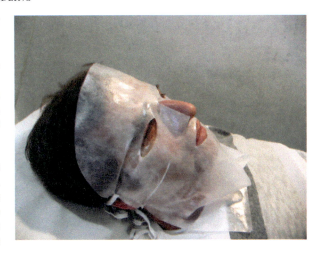

Figure 9.4 Application of a topical anesthetic (EMLA) on the facial skin in a patient affected with acne scars.

combination for treating scars and rejuvenating the skin, the number of needles on a roller is the least important feature, as repeated rolling causes numerous dermal injuries. Needle diameter is very important, as we are seeking to maximize the dermal injury without creating a new scar. In our experience, 0.25-mm needle diameter is of the maximum size that can be used without causing a new scar in the skin. Smaller diameter needle-skin rollers can be used but do not maximize the dermal injury and, therefore, will be slower to produce results.

Needle length is also a critical issue. The target when we needle the dermis is a layer in the upper dermis called the intermediate reticular dermis. This dermal layer contains the highest number of stem cells that are able to produce new collagen. The epidermis (the outer layer of the skin) varies in depth from .05 mm on the eyelids to 1.5 mm on the soles of the feet. The epidermis of the face (other than the eyelids) varies from 0.3 mm to 1 mm in depth and, therefore, a 0.75-mm to 2-mm-long needle is more than adequate to reach the intermediate reticular dermis. To treat acne scars, it is recommended that the professional device be used that is equipped with a rolling barrel 20 mm wide and 192 needles in 8 rows (Dermaroller model MF8; figure 9.5). The needles used should have a length of 1.5 mm and a diameter of 0.25 mm. Depending on the applied pressure (pressing too hard is not necessary for excellent results and if you are needling the face, do not use the rolling barrel on the eyelids or lips), they penetrate the scar tissue between 0.1 and 1.3 mm (Figure 9.6). Rolling consists in moving, with some pressure, 4 times in 4 directions: horizontally, vertically, and diagonally right and left (Figure 9.7). This ensure an even pricking pattern resulting in about 250 to 300 pricks per square centimeter. The microneedles penetrate through the epidermis but do not remove it; thus, the epidermis is only punctured and will rapidly heal. The needle seems to divide cells from each other rather than cutting through the cells so that many cells are spared.

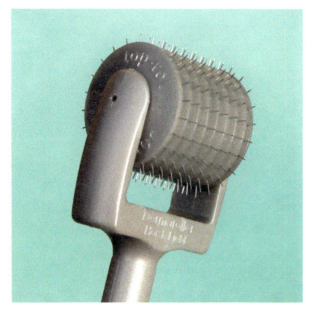

Figure 9.5 Dermaroller model MF8, by permission of Horst Leibl, Dermaroller, Fresenheim, France.

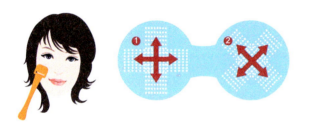

Figure 9.6 The professional device is rolled on the areas affected by acne scars in all possible directions.

MICRO SKIN NEEDLING

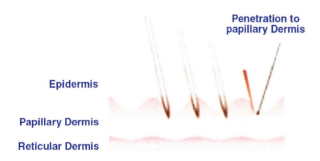

Figure 9.7 Micro Skin Needling.

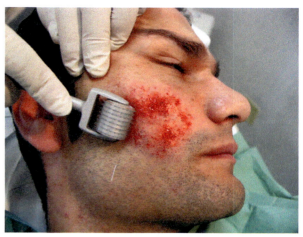

Figure 9.8 Bleeding.

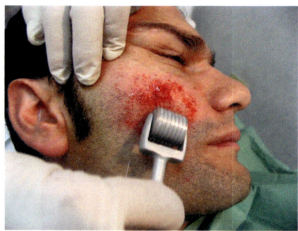

Figure 9.9 Bleeding.

Because the needles are set in a roller, every needle initially penetrates at an angle and then goes deeper as the roller turns. Finally, the needle is extracted at the converse angle; therefore, the tracts are curved, reflecting the path of the needle as it rolls into and then out of the skin, for about 1.3 mm into the dermis. The epidermis and particularly the stratum corneum remain "intact," except for these tiny holes, which are about four cells in diameter. The treatment times can range from 10 to 60 minutes, depending on the size of the area being treated. Naturally, the skin bleeds for a short time, but that soon stops (Figure 9.8–9.9). The skin develops multiple microbruises in the dermis that initiate the complex cascade of growth factors that eventually results in collagen production (Figure 9.10).

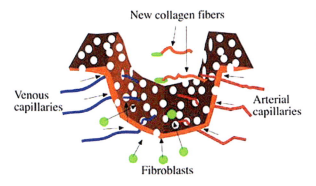

Figure 9.10 Schematic representation of collagen synthesis and angiogenesis induced by skin needling in an acne scar (from www.dermaroller.de, with permission).

POST-TREATMENT CARE

Postprocedure appearance (4) includes the following:

Day 1 and 2: Depending on how deeply the technician inserts the needle into the epidermis, the tissue may have slight to moderate swelling and may be tender, red, and bruised, with a slight lymph discharge from the treated areas. Minor itching may occur and the "needled" tissue may exhibit the appearance of "cat scratches."

Day 3: The treated areas slightly crust and remain faintly pink to red (Figure 9.11).

Day 4–5: The redness and crusting have diminished.

Day 5–7: There is barely any evidence of a procedure.

Healing time is 4 to 7 days and makeup can be worn after 2 to 3 days. Immediately after the treatment, the skin looks bruised, but bleeding is minimal, and there is only a small ooze of serum that soon stops (Figure 9.12). It's a good practice to apply cold compresses (no ice!) and vitamin-C mask. Some practitioners recommend soaking the skin with saline swabs for an hour or two and then cleaning the skin thoroughly with a oil-based cleanser. A thin layer of Vaseline or equivalent may be applied to reduce skin humidity loss. The patient is encouraged to use topical vitamin A and vitamin C as a cream or an oil to promote better healing and greater production of collagen. No products have to be applied on the treatment areas for 36 hours after treatment. Makeup and sunblock can be applied on Day 2 posttreatment, if the treatment area is dry and unbroken. Normal skincare can be recommended once the treatment area is completely healed. It is very important to continue using the topical vitamin cream for at least 6 months postprocedure to ensure the production of healthy collagen and elastin. The addition of peptides, like palmitoyl pentapeptide, could possibly ensure even better results. At home, the patient should stand under a shower for a long time, allowing the water to soak into the surface of the skin. Bathing is discouraged because of potential contamination from drains and plugs. Patients should be reminded to use only tepid water because the skin will be more sensitive to heat. While the water is running over the face or body, the patient should gently massage the treated skin until all serum,

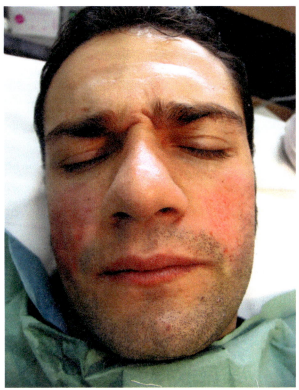

Figure 9.11 After the treatment the skin is reddened and swollen up to 3-4 days.

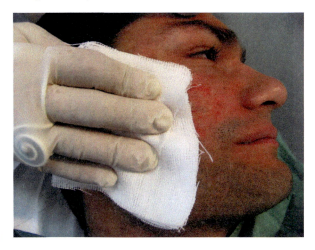

Figure 9.12 Bleeding and serum ooze rapidly stop by applying a sterile saline solution.

blood, or oil is removed. The importance of a thorough but gentle washing of the skin, a few hours after the procedure, cannot be stressed enough. The following day, the skin looks less dramatic and by Day 4 or 5, the skin has returned to a moderate pink flush, which can easily be concealed with makeup.

The patient should avoid direct sun exposure for at least 10 days, if possible, and use a broad-brimmed hat or scarf to protect the facial skin.

As the skin has a memory and will seek to return to its previous state, it's recommended to repeat skin-needling treatments over a period of 1 to 2 years. The outcome of collagen induction therapy combined with a prescribed posttreatment skin care routine can produce dramatic results that will last for years. So it's recommended that patients continue home needling to ensure the longevity of their scar improvement. The home needling can be safely combined with the use of peptide serum and/or tretinoin to maximize improvements in depressed scarring.

Results

Results generally start to be seen after about 6 weeks but the full effects can take at least 3 months to occur and, as the deposition of new collagen takes place slowly, the skin texture will continue to improve over a 12-month period. Clinical results vary between patients, with some achieving 90% improvement in scarring and others less than 50%. However, all patients achieve some improvements. The number of treatments (5) required varies depending on the individual collagen response on the condition of the tissue and desired results and will be determined by the dermatologist: You may need 2 to 6 treatments. Most individuals will require around 3 treatments approximately 4 weeks apart.

Our experience (6) has shown that, after only two sessions of treatment, the level of severity of rolling scars in all patients is largely reduced: The digital photographic comparison of lesions, before (Figure 9.13) and after CIT (Figure 9.14), highlighted that, (independently of the grading of lesions), in each group of patients, as skin became thicker, the relative rolling scar depth was significantly reduced. In fact, the Sign's Test for paired data (p value < 0.05) used to analyze the digital photographic data, highlights that the differences' median is negative, showing that the reduction of severity level of acne scars, before and after CIT, should be considered statistically significant. Moreover, the degree of irregularity of skin texture, while analyzing surface microrelief of cutaneous casts, showed a 25% reduction (average; in both axes) before (Figure 9.15) and after CIT (Figure 9.16). Besides, no patient showed visible signs of the procedure or hyperpigmentation.

Different studies report that 6 months after a collagen induction therapy a dramatic increase of new collagen and elastin fibers happens. Although difficult to estimate, there is at least 400% and 1000% more collagen and elastin in the postprocedure. Recently, Aust et al. showed a considerable increase in collagen and elastin deposition at 6 months postoperatively. The epidermis demonstrated 40% thickening of stratum spinosum and normal rete ridges at 1 year postoperatively.(7)

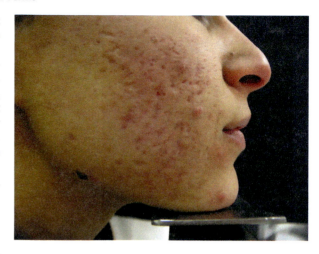

Figure 9.13 Facial acne scars in a female patient before skin needling.

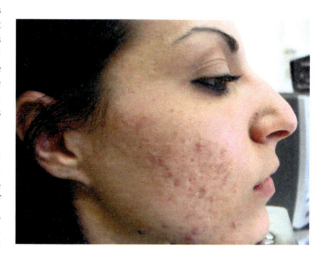

Figure 9.14 Facial acne scars in a female patient after skin needling.

MANAGEMENT OF COMPLICATIONS

- When the patient has not cleaned the skin thoroughly, a fine scab may form on the surface. The formation of scabs should be discouraged because they may cause obstruction and the development of simple milia or tiny pustules. Milia are uncommon, though, but when they occur they should be treated by pricking and draining. Tiny pustules are more common and usually found in patients treated for acne scars. It is important to open them early and make sure that the skin has been cleaned thoroughly and that there is no serous residue on the surface. When the pustules are allowed to dry on the skin, they will form thin scabs that effectively prevent the penetration of the vitamins necessary for a successful treatment.

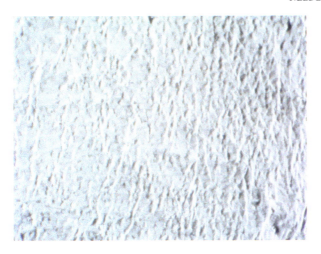

Figure 9.15 Surface microrelief of cutaneous casts from facial skin before skin needling.

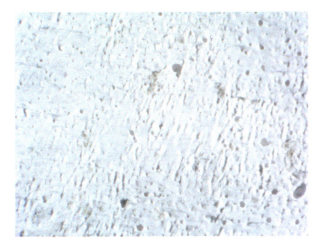

Figure 9.16 Surface microrelief of cutaneous casts from facial skin after skin needling: note the reduction of irregularity degree of skin texture.

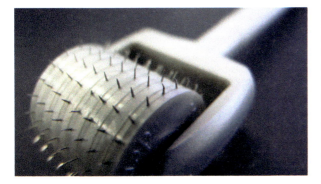

Figure 9.17 Professional device's micro-needles after acne scars' treatment: note how tips are bent like a fishhook.

- Herpes simplex is an uncommon complication, but if someone is prone to herpetic outbreaks, he or she needs to be on an antiviral medication prior to undergoing skin-needling procedure. Patients are instructed to use a topical virocidal if they feel the tingling feeling that is typical of herpes.
- After the skin has been needled, it becomes easier to penetrate, and much higher doses of vitamin A or alpha-hydroxiacid become available in the depth of the skin. Higher doses of vitamin A may cause a retinoid reaction that will aggravate the pink flush of the skin and also cause dry, flaky skin. A hydrating cream can be used to soothe the dry sensation.
- Overaggressive needling may cause scarring. This scarring does not seem to occur when using the special barrel of needles.
- Some medical devices can be autoclaved and stored for reuse for the same patient, but generally no longer than 6 months. In other cases, the medical device to be used is a disposable, single-use instrument: After an entire facial CIT-procedure, needles will loose their sharpness like any cutting devices, such as scalpels or razor blades, and it is recommended not to reuse the same device on the same patient. Moreover, it is absolutely recommended to not use badly tooled and copied version of the medical device: The material is too soft and the tips easily bend when touching a hard surface, for example, bones. The tips are bent like a fishhook (Figure 1.17). This again results in cutting and ripping tissue, nerves, vessels, and the lymphatic system when rolled through the skin. Most of these needles are too long: They prick and cut bigger subdermal vessels. This again results in severe and long-lasting hematomas (Figure 9.18). Also the possibility of a facial paralysis cannot be neglected.

FUTURE DEVELOPMENTS

Acne scarring is a difficult problem to be approached with a simple and definitive treatment solution. A combination of several treatment procedures may be appropriate, depending on specific patient features. Skin needling is a simple technique and can have an "immediate effect" on the improvement of rolling acne scars. In accordance with literature, a complete result after CIT may be observed after 8 to 12 months of treatment as the deposition of new collagen takes place slowly. As shown by D. Fernandes and M. Signorini, compared with the conventional methods, CIT has undisputable advantages. The most important one is that the epidermis remains intact because it is not damaged, eliminating most of the risks and negative side effects of chemical peeling or laser resurfacing. The skin needling and all its therapeutic possibilities are now being researched. There is scientific proof that the needling procedure also stimulates revascularization, repigments stretch marks, and fills cutaneous wrinkles. From this point of view, skin needling is now well established as a treatment option for depressed acne scarring because it is a procedure that is simple and fast and safely treats scars and is also a suitable procedure for different dermatologic pathologies.

SUMMARY

Skin needling is not an invasive and painful technique for acne scars treatment: It involves only a solicitation of skin surface, so as to ensure a fast recovery. Furthermore, it offers results not only comparable to other well-known procedures such as laser, chemical peeling, and dermabrasion but also faster healing.

REFERENCES

1. Orentreich DS, Orentreich N. Subcutaneous incisionless (subcision) surgery for the correction of depressed scars and wrinkles. Dermatol Surg 1995; 21: 543–9.
2. Fernandes D. Minimally invasive percutaneous collagen induction. Oral and Maxillofacial Surg Clin N Am 2005; 17: 51–63.
3. Liebl H. Abstract reflections about Collagen-Induction-Therapy (CIT). A hypothesis for the mechanism of action of collagen induction therapy (cit) using micro-needles, January 2–7. http://www.dermaroller.de/us/science/abstract-reflections-26.html February (accessed April 15 2009)."
4. Church S. Skin Needling - Natural Collagen Renewal. International Institute of Permanent Cosmetics. Internet paper.
5. McCaffrey P. Skin needling and rollers for scar reduction Australiahttp: //www.clearskincare.com.au/.
6. Fabbrocini G, Fardella N, Monfrecola A, Proietti I, Innocenzi D. Acne scarring treatment with skin needling. Clin Exp Derm 2008; in press.
7. Aust MC, Fernandes D, Kolokythas P et al. Percutaneous collagen induction therapy: an alternative treatment for scars, wrinkles, and skin laxity. Plast Reconstr Surg 2008; 121: 1421–9.

10 Fractional photothermolysis for acne scars
Kenneth R Beer

KEY FEATURES

- Acne scarring is a severe cosmetic concern for many adolescents as well as adults.
- Fractional photothermolysis treats only fractions of the skin.
- Several fractional laser devices are available and each varies as to the type of laser source, treatment settings, spot sizes, and treatment depth.
- The choice of which fractional device should be used is dependent on the type and depth of the scarring as well as the patient's skin type and tolerance for risk.
- Many new laser developments on the horizon including new fractional CO_2 laser systems require no anesthesia and are well tolerated.

INTRODUCTION

Fractional photothermolysis is a technology developed by Anderson and Manstein that removes fractions of the skin instead of wiping away the entire layer.(1) The benefits of fractional resurfacing include faster recovery time and lower rates of complications compared with traditional laser resurfacing. As with traditional laser resurfacing, different media may be utilized for fractional resurfacing. At the present time, the two most popular media for fractional resurfacing are carbon dioxide (CO_2) and erbium. Both target water and both vaporize the skin efficiently. The CO_2 laser penetrates to a deeper level than does erbium. These differences in depth of penetration have significant import with respect to the treatment of acne scars. Deeper scars may require the CO_2 fractional laser, while more superficial ones may be amenable to erbium.

Physicians have several options in regards to fractional laser systems, including ablative and non ablative laser systems. The depth and surface area of the scars being treated are the main determinants for system selection and energy settings. Ice-pick and deep acne scars are best treated with a fractional ablative laser able to penetrate deeper into the dermal depths where the abnormal, scarred collagen resides. Superficial scarring may be amenable to treatment with a fractional nonablative device. This less invasive device will improve the patient's appearance (and self-esteem) with less risk and minimal downtime. Additional treatment options for acne scars are available and the risks and benefits compared with fractional photothermolysis should be discussed with each patient prior to engaging in any type of treatment regimen. Chief among the options for the treatment of acne scars are dermabrasion, subcision, cosmetic fillers, chemical acid peels, punch biopsy, and excision.

ADVANTAGES OF FRACTIONAL LASERS FOR THE TREATMENT OF ACNE SCARS

Fractional photothermolysis offers many advantages when compared with traditional laser treatment of acne scars. Traditional CO_2 lasers were prone to many complications, including scarring, infection, and hyperpigmentation. This combination of sequelae were responsible for the decline in popularity of the procedure. When used for acne scars, the traditional CO_2 laser was able to improve some patient's scarring, but the potential to exacerbate the problem was significant. Traditional erbium lasers had lower rates of complications but were largely ineffective both for cosmetic indications and for the treatment of acne scarring. One publication that evaluated the outcomes of both CO_2 and erbium lasers for the treatment of acne scars concluded that most of the data that had been accumulated was insufficient to allow either patient or physician to conclude the degree to which traditional lasers improved acne scars.(2) Despite some publications and some physicians advocating the use of these lasers for the treatment of acne scars, the lack of data to support these claims led to the abandonment of the procedure for this indication. When these lasers became fractionated, the ability to treat acne scars once again became a subject of interest for physicians and surgeons alike.

HISTORY OF FRACTIONAL RESURFACING LASERS FOR THE TREATMENT OF ACNE SCARS

Since the technology of fractional thermolysis lasers is relatively new, the history of the use of these devices for this indication is short with few well-controlled clinical trials published prior to the publication of this book. The first publications regarding fractional laser technology came out in 2004 and the use of fractional laser technology for the treatment of acne scars began shortly thereafter.

A REVIEW OF SOME FRACTIONAL LASER DEVICES AND A REVIEW OF THEIR EFFICACY FOR THE TREATMENT OF ACNE SCARS

There are many different devices that may be utilized to treat acne scars. It is beyond the scope of this chapter to review the myriad devices that are used throughout the world. Instead, a focus will be placed on the systems that are most prevalent at the present time. Although the various manufacturers incorporate different technologies and have differences in their treatment algorithms, some general trends are valid across the various platforms. It will be useful to have an understanding of the present fractional laser devices as indicated for the treatment of acne scars.

The first widely available fractional laser was introduced by Reliant and was known as the Fraxel. A Medline search of

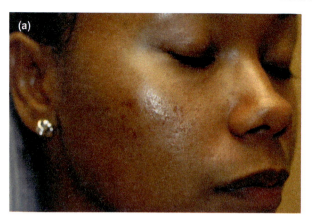
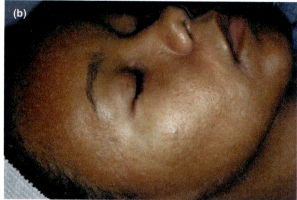

Figure 10.1 (A) Moderate acne scars in a common location, the cheeks. The patient is a type VI skin type. (B) Following three treatments with the Fraxel 1550 laser, the appearance of the scars is improved. There is no evidence of any hyperpigmentation. (Courtesy of Dr. Jill Waibel.)

fractional laser treatment of acne scars reveals that this is also the device that has been most widely used in publications reporting treatment of acne scars with fractional lasers. This device uses an erbium source at a wavelength of 1550.(3) Early versions of this required the use of a blue dye to enable the tracking system to scan the areas that had and had not been treated. This was viewed by many as an inconvenience and subsequent devices no longer use this dye. Typical configurations of the Fraxel laser incorporate a chilling device from Zimmer to cool the skin as the laser treats it. This cooling has several functions but the two most relevant ones for the treatment of acne scars is that it enables the patient to tolerate higher energy levels, thereby reaching depths typical of acne scars. A second advantage is theoretical, but it is possible that this chilling protects the bulge portion of the hair follicle enabling the stem cells to repopulate the skin from a deeper (and thus more even) level.

Fraxel lasers enable the physician to alter the depth and density of the beamlets. When treating acne, this ability allows the user to increase the density when it is necessary to ablate more of the surface area and to increase the depth (energy) to treat deeper scars. Whereas other techniques such as dermabrasion and chemical peeling do not enable the physician to match the depth of the treatment to the depth of the acne scar, Fraxel can alter the depth of penetration to precisely accomplish this. Thus, at an energy setting of 20 mJ, the depth of the laser penetration is 794 μ, while at 40 mJ it is 1120 μ.(4) As with any system, one limitation is that treatments are uncomfortable at high-energy settings so the use of topical or injectional anesthetic is beneficial.

In clinical experience, the Fraxel has been used to treat acne scars with a high degree of patient satisfaction for scars that are relatively small and relatively shallow (Figure 10.1). One study that evaluated the use of the initial model of this laser to treat mild-to-moderate atrophic acne scars in 53 patients concluded that the treatments were safe and effective.(5) Acne scars in this study were treated monthly for 3 months. The authors found that clinical improvements in the range of 51% to 75% were seen in nearly all (90%) of the subjects treated. Few complications were noted. Whether additional treatments would have improved scars to a greater extent or intrinsic collagen remodeling helped diminish the appearance of the scars after the study concluded is not known.

The Fraxel SR model is an improved device that does not require the use of blue dyes to target the laser. This has also been demonstrated to improve the appearance of acne scars. Chrastil et al. evaluated the Fraxel SR for the treatment of acne scars in skin types I–V. The SR model enabled treatments at higher fluences and greater densities than prior models. Fluences used in these patients were between 35–40 mJ/ microthermal zone and the percent of treatment coverage was between 20% and 35%. Following between two and six treatments, the majority of patients had an improvement in the appearance of their acne scars between 50% and 75%.(6) These authors also noted no adverse events with the use of this device to treat acne scars.

Many different skin types have been treated with this device in an effort to treat acne scars. Acne scars in types V and VI skin are notoriously difficult to treat with many treatment regimens resulting in hyperpigmentation, hypopigmentation, and keloid formation. Fraxel treatment of 27 patients with types V and VI skin were performed to treat moderate-to-severe acne scars. In these patients, 30% of patients reported excellent improvements, while another 50% reported significant improvement. As with other reports, adverse events were limited to transient issues such as erythema and edema. The authors concluded that fractional resurfacing (Fraxel) was a significantly effective means of treating acne scars in this patient population.(7)

One fractional CO_2 laser with the ability to penetrate deeply and treat acne scars is the UltraPulse from Lumenis. This device

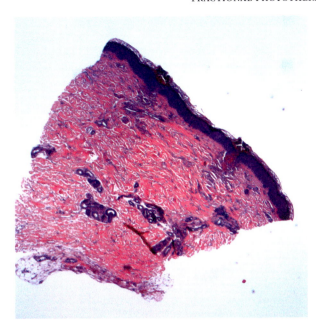

Figure 10.2 Fractional CO_2 laser using the Lumenis Ultrapulse. This biopsy demonstrates the ability of fractional CO_2 lasers to penetrate to the depth of the acne scar as well as its ability to spare the intervening tissue. It is this latter property that enables rapid healing.

has been engineered to deliver higher energy levels than many other devices on the market with peak energy levels of 225 mJ. It combines two different modalities, Deep FX and Active FX, to enable the physician to address superficial and deep acne scars. One characteristic of the device that lends itself to the treatment of acne scars is its limited thermal spread due to its short pulse duration of <1 ms. This device is also able to treat deep scars with the Deep FX hand piece, which penetrates deeper into the skin (Figure 10.2); the Active FX hand piece may be used to treat superficial scarring. This laser also has a large scan pattern size of up to 10 mm × 10 mm, enabling the physician to treat large body surfaces in a relatively short amount of time. This device affords better results as seen with traditional CO_2 lasers with a decreased recovery time and, therefore, increased patient satisfaction. Currently a study is being done to determine the recovery rate of patients treated with the Active FX in comparison with traditional CO_2 resurfacing techniques[h1] [h1] [h1].(8)

Fractional photothermolysis has been used to treat patients who had a combination of mild-to-moderate acne scars combined with enlarged pores.(9) This population is representative of many patients presenting for treatment. The system used for this trial was a Lutronic 1,550 nm erbium glass laser. A total of 12 patients with type V skin were treated with 3 sessions spaced 1 month apart. Improvement was evaluated by a blinded

observer who concluded that 8 patients had improvements of between 51% and 100% in 4 months after the last treatment was performed. Complications seen during the study were limited to treatment related erythema and swelling. No significant hyperpigmentation or scarring was noted. This study was notable for demonstrating histology associated with the treatment, and it is notable for demonstrating isolated microthermal zone damage to the epidermis and collagen. The depth of the injury is comparable to the depth associated with many mild-to-moderate acne scars, and it is possible that this correlation of treatment depth to the underlying pathophysiology of the acne scar is responsible for the high degree of improvement. The depth did not appear to be deep enough to ablate the hair matrix, and this probably is the reason why scarring was avoided. In this study, patient satisfaction was more correlated with improvement of acne scars than with pore size

Fractional photothermolysis lasers are made by many companies. Each device has strengths and weaknesses that have important implications for treating acne scars. Differences in the lasers include different wavelengths, spot sizes, fluence levels, density of laser beamlets, skin cooling systems, and ease of use (for both physician and patient). Another critical difference for the treatment of acne scars is the degree to which the different devices have been used in well-designed clinical trials. As with any indication, it is important to have a reasonable likelihood of success with good patient safety profile.

Slim Evolution Lasering recently developed a microspot system with a fractional modality (Mixto SX). This new function prolongs the time between two adjacent treatment spots. This modality prevents heat from building up around the treated spots, thus significantly reducing pain throughout the treatment. With fractional photothermolysis, some form of topical anesthesia and/or cooling system is needed. With the Mixto SX, the procedure is well tolerated without any anesthesia or skin-cooling system.(10) The Mixto SX laser system also has the traditional single CO_2 laser beam that can be used to remove solid lesions or to make incisions. This setting can be switched with the touch of a button and no need to swap handpieces. Patients with acne scars can be treated with such a laser, and because no anesthesia or cooling is needed, it decreases the time in office.

Palomar also makes a fractional erbium laser. It uses a wavelength of 1,540 nm and also targets water as the chromophore. In addition to these two devices, the Affirm, a 1,440 nm Nd:Yag fractional laser produced by Cynosure (Westford, MA), the ProFractional made by Sciton (Palo Alto, CA), Ultrapulse manufactured by Lumenis (Santa Clara, CA), the Juvia by Ellipse (Atlanta, GA), and many other devices may be used for fractional laser treatments of acne scars. There are many significant differences between the various laser systems. The differences, some subtle others not so subtle, have significant bearing on their use for esthetic rejuvenation in general and the treatment of acne scars in particular.

From the perspective of the physician using the device, the most significant difference between various devices is whether it is ablative or not. Ablative devices use CO_2 and penetrate to a deeper level than do nonablative systems. The degree of collagen stimulation from the ablative devices will be significantly more compared to that of a nonablative device utilized. For acne scars, deeper and broader scars may be treated effectively with ablative devices capable of resurfacing to a deeper level. More superficial acne scars, requiring less depth for scar correction, need nonablative erbium lasers.

Considerations other than whether a device is ablative or nonablative are also important for treating acne scars. Some machines have scanners that allow the operator to dial in the depth, while some others use energy settings as a proxy for depth. When treating acne scars, it is helpful to have the ability to match the depth of resurfacing to the depth of the scar. Many devices have fixed-spot sizes that are larger than the scars being treated. This requires the user to manually calculate the depth needed.

Whereas the Palomar system has a fixed-spot size that must be manually moved to stamp out the treated areas, the Reliant system uses a handpiece that uses rollers to scan across the skin. This enables the physician to focus on certain locations. In this case, treating acne scars means that instead of treating the areas around the scar, the laser may be used to treat the scar itself and blur the boundaries between it and adjacent, normal skin. Acne scars are notoriously variable in their depth, which is one reason why they are so prominent. The Reliant fractional device enables the user to change the depth of the beam with a great degree of precision so that the laser can approximate the depth of the scar.

CO_2 fractional lasers are also available from Reliant, and these devices may be useful for treating deeper acne scars. These devices deliver a 30 W CO_2 laser light at a wavelength of 10,600 nm. In comparison with nonablative fractional devices, ablative fractionals utilize the same concept of treating only microscopic areas that are then surrounded by healthy untreated skin. With only a portion of the skin treated, the patient will experience less perioperative discomfort and decreased postoperative complications. The novelty of CO_2 fractional laser is that it enables better outcomes as seen with traditional CO_2 lasers, but with less downtime and adverse effects.

According to Zachary et al., acne scarring is most common "on the mid cheek and temple area".(11) Acneiform scars are a result of damage to collagen production in the deep dermal layers.(12) In patients with superficial or moderate acne scars, treatment with fractional lasers may produce dramatic results. However, those with deep, depressed acne scars with sharp borders may not respond well to fractional resurfacing and may require other modalities such as excisions, chemical peels, or a combination of modalities. One interesting possibility is the combined use of fillers such as hyaluronic acid with fractional resurfacing. The hyaluron would lift the deep portion of the scar up and reduce the volume of scar, while the fractional laser would blur the borders of the epidermal components. Several other combinations of fillers (including the use of porcine collagen) with fractional lasers may yield results not obtainable with technique alone and research into optimizing these combinations is warranted. Additional possible adjuncts discussed elsewhere in this text may be combined with fractional laser resurfacing to improve the appearance of acne scars.

OUTLOOK AND FUTURE DEVELOPMENTS
Research into the use of fractional photothermolysis (both ablative and nonablative) is being conducted for the treatment of a variety of scars. Whereas the etiology of scars that result from burns and scars resulting from acne have differing pathophysiology, it is likely that the use of these lasers for each will yield insights into ways to help the other. A better understanding of the molecular biology underlying the remodeling of collagen, elastin, and the epidermis, following treatment with fractional photothermolysis, will indubitably result in means to enhance the outcomes for laser treatments for acne scars. Combinations of surface-scanning laser imaging married to fractional thermolysis that is directed toward individual scars has the potential to customize fractional laser treatments for acne scars with potential increased efficacy. Finally, as the lasers themselves become more technologically advanced, it is inevitable that they will be used for better effect to treat this prevalent and disfiguring problem.

SUMMARY FOR THE CLINICIAN
Fractional lasers offer effective treatment for many types of acne scars. They may be used at depths that match the depth of the scars in question.

Both ablative and nonablative lasers have a role in the treatment of acne scars, and choosing between the two requires a knowledge of the differences between them, the depths of the scars, and an understanding of the interaction of these devices with different skin types.

REFERENCES
1. Manstein D, Herron GS, Sink RK, Tanner H, Anderson RR. Fractional photothermolysis: a new concept for cutaneous remodeling using microscopic patterns of thermal injury. Lasers Surg Med 2004; 34(5): 426–38.
2. Jordan R. Cummins C, Burls A. Laser resurfacing of the skin for the improvement of facial acne scarring: a systematic review of the evidence. Br J Dermatol 2000; 142: 413–23.
3. Pubmed accessed on Nov. 22, 2008.
4. Source: Reliant Inc. Hawyard CA.
5. Alster T, Tanzi E and Lazarus M. The use of fractional laser photothermolysis for the treatment of atrophic scars. Dermatol Surg 2007; 33: 295–9.
6. Chrastil B, Glaich AS, Goldberg LH, Friedman PM. Second generation 1,550 nm fractional photothermolysis for the treatment of acne scars. Dermatol Surg 2008; 34(10): 1327–32.
7. Lee HS, Lee JH, Ahn GY et al. Fractional photothermolysis for the treatment of acne scars: a report of 27 Korean Patients. J Dermatolog Treat 2008; 19(1): 45–9.

8. Goldberg, David. Reduced Down-time associated with novel fractional ultrapulse CO_2 treatment (ActiveFX) as compared to traditional CO_2 resurfacing. JAAD 2007; 56(2): AB206.

9. Cho SB, Lee JH, Choi MJ, Lee KY, Oh SH. Efficacy of the fractional photothermolysis system with dynamic operating mode on acne scars and enlarged pores. Dermatol Surg 2009; 35: 108–14.

10. Cassuto D. An innovative device for fractional CO_2 laser resurfacing: a preliminary clinical study. Am J Cosmet Surg 2008; 25(2): 97–101.

11. Zachary C, Rokhsar C, Fitzpatrick R. Laser Skin Resurfacing in Goldberg D. Lasers and Lights Vol II.

12. Chapas AM, Brightman L, Sukal S et al. Successful treatment of acne scars w/CO_2. Lasers Surg Med 2008; 40(6): 381–6.

11   Nonablative and ablative devices for the treatment of acne scars
Vic A Narurkar

INTRODUCTION
Acne scars are polymorphous and require a multidimensional approach to successful treatments. Scars can be atrophic, hypertrophic, sharply marginated, incongruous, distensible, and nondistensible. Surface anomalies could include erythema, hypopigmentation, and hyperpigmentation. The advent of lasers, light sources, and radiofrequency has added significantly to the treatment and management of postacne scarring. It is imperative to understand the indications for the class of devices to create a successful algorithm in incorporating devices for the treatment of postacne scarring. This chapter will review the various light sources, nonablative and ablative lasers, and radiofrequency devices for acne scarring.

FLASH LAMP PULSED-DYE LASER (FPDL) AT 585 NM AND 595 NM
The FPDL was one of the first lasers utilized to treat hypertrophic and erythematous scars.(1, 2) The primary target of the FPDL is oxyhemoglobin. Therefore, the primary objective of using this device is to improve the erythema, which is often prominent in early acne scars. In addition to erythema, improvement in texture of scars has been observed, leading to the hypothesis that a nonablative mode of dermal remodeling and collagen production is involved. Higher fluencies of FPDL are indicated for hypertrophic scars and lower fluencies for atrophic scars. The FPDL has also shown to have a coincidental improvement of active acne, although this has been a hotly debated topic. The mechanisms for acne clearance involve collateral damage to sebaceous glands and destruction of *Propionobacterium* acnes. Transforming growth factor Beta 1 mRNA has been shown to increase in patients after FPDL treatments. TGF-beta is known to be a potent stimulus for neocollagenesis and also promotes resolution of inflammation, which may explain the dual benefits of FPDL in active acne resolution/erythema resolution and long-term improvement in acne scars. Three to five sessions with FPDL spaced 4 to 6 weeks apart are usually necessary (Figure 11.1).

BROADBAND LIGHT SOURCES WITH FILTERS (INTENSE PULSED LIGHT)
Broadband light uses selective filters, the majority of which are in the visible light range. Hence, it was appropriate to utilize these devices in a similar manner to the FPDL for the nonablative treatment of acne scarring.(3) As with FPDL, 3 to 5 treatment sessions are usually necessary and the indications are similar to those with FPDL-primarily subtle, atrophic, and hypertrophic scars, with the primary goal being improvement of visible erythema. Coincidental improvement of active acne has also been reported.

PHOTOPNEUMATIC THERAPY
Photopneumatic therapy utilizes lower wavelength photons in the 420- to 500-nm range as a broadband light source compared to traditional visible light filters in broadband light.(4) Concurrent vacuum is applied at the time of light delivery, allowing for dermal targets to be closer to the surface, allowing for more efficient light delivery. These devices primarily treat active acne, as the target is *Propionobacterium* acnes. Subtle improvements in shallow nondistensible and erythematous scars, similar to those with FPDL and IPL are also seen (Figure 11.2). It is also possible that stretching the skin with the vacuum may create some mechanical forces that may lead to long-term dermal remodeling.

LONG-PULSED 1,064 NM LASERS
The long-pulsed 1,064 nm lasers were originally developed for hair reduction in darker skin tones. Coincidental improvement in skin texture and tone were observed in hair reduction patients, leading physicians to utilize these lasers for the treatment of postacne scarring. The primary chromophore for the LP 1,064 nm laser is water, with some absorption by hemoglobin, although significantly less than that by FPDL and IPL sources. Therefore, similar to the other nonablative devices, the LP 1,064 is also indicated for subtle improvement of distensible nonerythematous acne scars.(5, 6) The inherent wavelength of these devices also makes them a better option in treating darker skin tones. It is imperative to utilize lower fluencies and excellent cooling with these devices, as higher fluencies and poor cooling could actually promote scarring. Histology shows neocollagenesis, similar to that seen with other nonablative devices. Treatment intervals are 2 to 4 weeks apart and necessitate 3 to 5 treatment sessions.

Q-SWITCHED 1,064 NM LASERS
The Q switched 1,064 nm lasers employ an optomechanical shutter allowing for nanosecond delivery of laser pulses at the 1,064 nm wavelength. The laser was originally developed for the treatment of decorative tattoos of blue black ink. The mechanism of tattoo removal is primarily photoacoustic, while the mechanism for dermal remodeling for acne scars is a combination of photoacoustic effects and absorption by water, leading to dermal collagen remodeling.(7) This is the safest laser in darker skin tones and does not require contact cooling. Lower fluencies are indicated for acne scarring, in comparison with decorative tattoo removal. Three to five treatment sessions, spaced 4 to 6 weeks apart, are necessary.

1,320 NM LASER
The 1,320 nm was the first laser to be studied specifically for nonablative resurfacing of rhytids. The mechanism was to

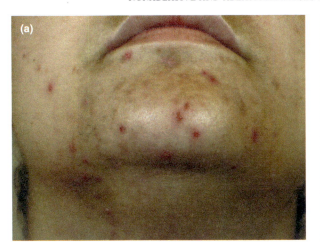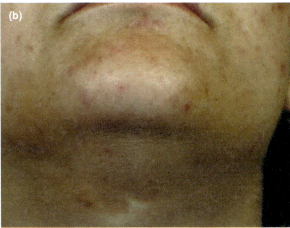

Figure 11.1 Distensible erythematous acne scars (A) before and (B) after 3 treatments with 585 nm Flash-lamped, pulsed-dye laser.

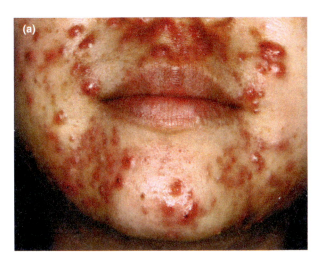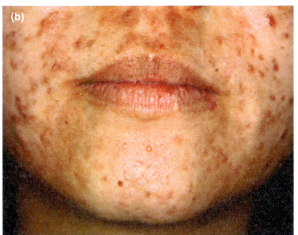

Figure 11.2 Concurrent improvement of active acne and distensible erythematous acne scars (A) before and (B) after five treatments with photopneumatic therapy.

utilize the 1,320 nm wavelength, which has deep penetration into the dermis, bypassing the epidermis and protecting the epidermis with cryogen cooling. The results with rhytids have generally been disappointing, but the results with nondistensible acne scarring have been better.(8)

1,450 NM DIODE LASER
As with the 1,320 nm laser, the 1,450 nm diode laser was originally developed for nonablative resurfacing of rhytids. A coincidental observation of the 1,450 nm laser was its effect on the sebaceous gland, causing thermal necrosis.(9) Hence, lesions of active acne vulgaris improved after a series of treatments. The nonselective absorption of water and the deeper penetration permitted the concurrent dermal remodeling and neocollagenesis, allowing

this laser to also be utilized for scarring. The deeper penetration allowed for the treatment of more significant scarring, unlike some of the other nonablative devices such as FPDL, IPL, and 1,064 nm lasers. Atrophic as well as flat and hypertrophic scars can be treated successfully. A series of 3 to 5 treatments, spaced 4 to 6 weeks apart, is indicated. The concurrent improvement of acne is also a bonus. The main limiting factor of the 1,450 nm diode laser is the significant discomfort, necessitating the use of strong topical anesthetics.

1,540 NM AND 1,550 NM NONABLATIVE FRACTIONAL LASERS
The most significant advance in the treatment of acne scarring is the development of nonablative fractional laser resurfacing

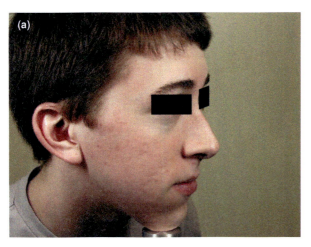 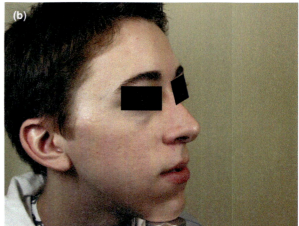

Figure 11.3 Polymorphous acne scars (A) before and (B) after 5 treatments with 1,550 nm nonablative fractional laser resurfacing.

in the mid-infrared region.(10, 11) These lasers were originally developed for skin resurfacing for photodamage because ablative laser resurfacing had significant risks while nonablative laser resurfacing produced minimal results. While these lasers offer excellent result in resurfacing for mild-to-moderate photodamage, the most impressive results are seen with postacne scarring. The chromophore is water and the depth of penetration is up to 1 mm and beyond in the dermis. The laser energy is delivered in a fractional array of microbeams, either in a stamped fashion (1,540 nm laser) or a random pattern (1,550 nm). The fractional mode of delivery creates microscopic areas of injury. Treatment densities and fluencies can be adjusted based on the extent of acne scarring, anatomic location, and skin tone. All skin colors can be treated with safety. The fractional mode of energy delivery reduces bulk heating, which has been the major source of complications in both ablative and nonablative lasers. All types of acne scars—ice pick, rolling, boxcars, distensible, nondistensible, and erythematous—can be treated successfully (Figure 11.3). Moreover, hypopigmented scars can also be treated successfully with nonablative fractional laser resurfacing. The need for adjuvant treatments of ice-pick and bound-down scars (e.g., subcision) has been reduced considerably since the advent of fractional laser resurfacing. Three to seven sessions, spaced 4 to 6 weeks apart, are indicated.

ABLATIVE 2,940 AND 10,600 NM FRACTIONAL LASERS
The development of ablative 2,940 nm and 10,600 nm lasers (12) was promoted due to the need of fewer treatments in skin resurfacing compared with nonablative lasers and to reduce risks with traditional ablative laser resurfacing at these wavelengths. These devices are relatively new and there are limited data on the efficacy with acne scarring. The 2,940 nm wavelength shows the greatest affinity for water,

but with higher fluencies needed for ablation, still produces greater bleeding. The 10,600 nm wavelength is best utilized with higher fluencies, allowing for deeper penetration. There have been some reports of impressive improvements with the fractional 10,600 nm ablative laser for acne scars with fewer treatments than with the nonablative fractional lasers.(13)

TRADITIONAL 2,940 NM AND 10,600 NM ABLATIVE LASERS
Traditional ablative laser resurfacing employs 2,940 nm or 10,600 nm wavelengths. These devices have lost popularity due to prolonged healing and recovery, and with the case of 10,600 nm ablative laser resurfacing, outcomes reveal significant risks of hypopigmentation. The traditional 10,600 nm ablative laser offered advantages over the traditional 2,940 nm ablative laser because of greater hemostasis. The advent of longer pulsed 2,940 nm lasers now can produce better hemostasis. For acne scarring, the ablative 2,940 nm may offer advantages over 10,600 nm because of deeper penetration, thereby allowing the treatment of a wider variety of acne scars.(14, 15)

COMBINATION THERAPIES
Table 11.1 summarizes the monotherapy approach for the treatment of acne scars. It is evident that, as with facial rejuvenation, the approach to acne scarring requires a multimodal approach. This is especially true for ice-pick scars, deep scars, and communicating scars. Punch excision is often necessary if scars are extensive and ice pick in nature, although the need for this has been considerably reduced with the advent of nonablative fractional laser resurfacing. Subcision is indicated when scars are bound down and have communicating sinus tracts. Dermal fillers are indicated when there is still atrophy despite treatment with devices.

Table 11.1 Summary of Laser and Light Based Devices for Acne Scars.

Device	Mode	Type of Acne Scars for Optimal Treatment
585 nm, 595 nm Flash lamp pulsed-dye laser	Nonablative	Erythematous and distensible scars
Broadband light; Photopneumatic therapy	Nonablative	Erythematous, hyperpigmented, and distensible scars
Long pulsed 1,064 nm laser	Nonablative	Distensible acne scars; subtle pitted scars
Q switched 1,064 nm laser	Nonablative	Distensible acne scars; subtle pitted scars
1,320 nm laser	Nonablative	Distensible acne scars; subtle-to-moderate pitted and boxcar scars
1,450 nm laser	Nonablative	Distensible acne scars; subtle-to-moderate pitted and boxcar scars
1,540 nm & 1,550 nm lasers	Fractional nonablative	Polymorphous scars
2,940 nm & 10,600 nm lasers	Fractional ablative	Polymorphous scars
2,940 nm & 10,600 nm lasers	Ablative	Polymorphous scars

CONCLUSIONS

A variety of devices are successful in treating postacne scarring. The nonablative devices include the FPDL, IPL, LP 1,064 nm laser, QS 1,064 nm laser, 1,320 nm laser, and 1,450 nm laser. These nonablative devices are best for subtle shallow acne scarring and acne-associated erythema. The 1,320 nm and 1,450 nm may offer additional benefits for more extensive scarring. The nonablative fractional lasers include the 1,540 nm and 1,550 nm laser and are considered the gold standard for acne scarring, treating the widest variety of polymorphous acne scars and diminishing the need for punch excisions and subcisions. The ablative fractional lasers include the 2,940 nm and 10,600 nm lasers, which have been introduced more recently and may offer results similar to that derieved using nonablative fractional lasers, but with fewer treatments. Traditional ablative lasers include the 2,940 nm and 10,600 nm lasers, and, though effective for treating postacne scarring, lead to both significant recovery and risks. Devices are best employed in acne scarring, using a combination of subcision, punch excisions, and dermal fillers for complete treatment.

REFERENCES

1. Railan D, Alster TS. Laser treatment of acne, psoriasis, leukoderma and scars. Semin Cutan Med Surg 2008; 27(4): 285–91.
2. Lee DH, Choi YS, Min SU, Yoon MY, Suh DH. Comparison of 585 nm pulsed dye laser and a 1,064 nm Nd:YAG laser for the treatment of acne scars: a randomized split faced study. J Am Acad Dermatol 2009; 60(5): 801–7.
3. Sawcer D, Lee HR, Lowe NJ. Lasers and adjunctive treatments for facial scars: a review. J Cutan Laser Ther 1999; 1(2): 77–85.
4. Shamban AT, Enokibori M, Narurkar V, Wilson D. Photopneumatic technology for the treatment of acne vulgaris. J Drugs Dermatol 2008; 7(2): 139–45.
5. Keller R, Belda Junior W, Valente NY, Rodrigues CJ. Nonablative 1,064 nm Nd:YAG laser resurfacing of facial atrophic acne scars: histologic and clinical analysis. Dermatol Surg 2007; 33(12): 1470–6.
6. Goldberg DJ. Nonablative laser surgery for pigmented skin. Dermatol Surg 2005; 31(10): 1263–7.
7. Friedman PM, Jih MH, Skover GR et al. Treatment of facial atrophic scars with the 1,064 nm Q-switched Nd:YAG laser-six month follow up study. Arch Dermatol 2004; 140(11): 1337–41.
8. Yaghmai D, Garden JM, Bakus AD, Massa MC. Comparison of a 1,064 nm laser and a 1,320 nm laser for the nonablative treatment of acne scars. Dermatol Surg 2005; 31: 903–9.
9. Chua SH, Ang P, Khoo LS, Goh CL. Nonablative 1,450 nm diode laser in the treatment of facial atrophic scars in type IV to V Asian skin: a prospective clinical study. Dermatol Surg 2004; 30(10): 1287–91.
10. Narurkar V. Skin rejuvenation with microthermal fractional photothermolysis. Dermatol Ther 2007; 20(Suppl 1): S10–3.
11. Taub AF. Fractionated delivery systems for difficult to treat clinical applications: acne scarring, melasma, atrophic scarring, striae distensae and deep rhytides. J Drugs Dermatol 2007; 6(11): 1120–8.
12. Geronemus RG. Fractional photothermolysis: current and future applications. Lasers Surg Med 2006; 38(3): 169–76.
13. Chapas AM, Brightman L, Sukal S et al. Successful treatment of acneiform scarring with CO2 ablative fractional resurfacing. Lasers Surg Med 2008; 40(6): 381–6.
14. Jeong JT, Kye YC. Resurfacing of pitted facial acne scars with a long pulsed Er:YAG laser. Dermatol Surg 2001; 27(2): 107–10.
15. Walia S, Alster TS. Prolonged clinical and histologic effects from CO2 laser resurfacing of atrophic acne scars. Dermatol Surg 1999; 25(12): 926–30.

12 Surgical techniques: Excision, grafting, punch techniques, and subcision
Megan Pirigyi and Murad Alam

KEY FEATURES

- Treatment approaches for acne scarring should be individualized and primarily determined by the particular morphological features of each patient's scars.
- The surgical interventions described in this chapter are indispensable in the revision of deep and fibrotic acne scars.
- Subcision is a simple, well-tolerated procedure capable of producing long-term improvement of rolling acne scars.
- Dermal grafts are autologous implants that may provide permanent augmentation of depressed acne scars.
- Excision and punch techniques remain the treatments of choice for deep, sharply punched-out acne scars.
- All the procedures described in this chapter may be incorporated into multistep treatment plans tailored to address patients' individual needs.

INTRODUCTION

The problem of acne scarring cannot be solved by a single "best" treatment. Acne scars come in a wide variety of structures and depths, and each of the currently available treatments is ideally suited to address a subset of this spectrum. While resurfacing procedures are useful in resolving texture and pigment irregularities caused by shallow to medium-depth acne scars, fillers may be effective in augmenting depressed, distensible scars. The surgical interventions described in this chapter, including excision, punch techniques, subcision, and dermal grafting, are often the best available options for improving the deepest and most fibrotic forms of acne scarring.

The common objective of all excision and punch techniques is to replace deep, sharply delineated scars, such as ice-pick and deep boxcar scars, with less conspicuous secondary defects. In elliptical and punch excision, this is accomplished by surgical removal of a scar and careful closure of the resultant defect to create a flat, linear scar that lies along a relaxed skin-tension line. Punch grafting entails replacing an excised scar with a full-thickness, autologous punch graft, and punch elevation involves preserving an excised scar base and allowing it to rise to the level of the surrounding skin.

Both subcision and dermal grafting are aimed at achieving long-term augmentation of depressed acne scars with indistinct borders. Subcision, or subdermal undermining, is designed to treat rolling acne scars resulting from abnormal fibrous tethering of scar surfaces to deeper structures. Because of their underlying physiology, these scars are not amenable to correction by fillers alone but may be improved when subcision is used to disrupt the fibrous bands below their surfaces. Dermal grafting involves implantation of an autologous strip or plug of dermis into a subcised recipient pocket and may achieve long-term augmentation of deeper depressed scars caused by dermal loss.

For all of the surgical techniques described in this chapter, careful patient selection and ongoing communication are paramount. While these procedures have the potential to improve the appearance of some of the most severe forms of acne scarring, patients must have realistic expectations about the degree of improvement they are likely to achieve. Although irregularities in contour, texture, and pigmentation may be ameliorated, complete erasure of a scar is highly unlikely. Since many patients have a variety of different acne scar types and because some of these treatments involve the creation of secondary defects, a combination of different procedures over the course of many months is often required to produce optimal results. In addition, when designing a treatment strategy one should carefully consider a patient's willingness to accept downtime. Before recommending any scar revision procedures, it is crucial to obtain a thorough medical and surgical history. Patients with increased risk of keloid and hypertrophic scarring and those with active or newly resolved acne are not good candidates for surgical scar revision.[1] (Table 12.1)

Table 12.1 Patient characteristics that are possible contraindications for surgical scar treatment.

Characteristic	Reason for Contraindication
History of poor wound healing or tendency toward keloid formation/hypertrophic scarring	Risk of unacceptable secondary defect
Unreasonable expectations for improvement	Complete elimination of a scar is highly unlikely. Optimal results may require a combination of treatment modalities over the course of several months.
Active or recently resolved acne lesions	Disruption of pilosebaceous units during surgical procedures may lead to formation of acneiform cysts

SUBCISION

History

In 1995, Orentreich and Orentreich introduced the technique of subcision as a stand-alone treatment for depressed scars and wrinkles.(2) However, the technique of subdermal undermining of scars has been used since as early as 1957, when it was described as a method to prepare sites for fibrin foam injection. (3) Since that time, undermining has been used frequently in conjunction with fibrel implantation, (4, 5) microlipoinjection, (6) and dermal grafting (7) procedures.

Structure and Function

Subcision is designed to address the underlying pathophysiology of rolling acne scars. These scars appear as broad, undulating depressions on the surface of the skin and lack the sharply delineated edges seen in boxcar and icepick scars. Despite their superficial appearance, rolling scars result from deep fibrous attachments tethering the epidermis to the subcutis. Subcision is designed to sever these fibrous bands while causing minimal damage to the overlying skin. Ideally, this technique results in elevation of the depressed scar to the level of the surrounding skin. The originators of this technique, David and Norman Orentreich, propose that subcision's augmenting effect is achieved by two distinct processes.(2) An immediate, partial elevation results from the scar base being cut free from the downward pull of its tethers.(2, 8) In the weeks following subcision, additional augmentation of the depressed defect is typically observed. This subsequent elevation is thought to result from trauma caused during the procedure, which initiates a wound-healing response culminating in the deposition of new connective tissue beneath the scar surface.(2, 9)

Technology

Indication

This technique is best used to treat rolling acne scars with normal-appearing overlying skin and a lack of sharply delineated borders.(2) It is contraindicated for areas of active infection and in patients with bleeding diathesis or a tendency toward keloid formation.(2) Other cutaneous depressions, such as rhytids, depressed skin grafts, surgical wounds, and cellulite dimples are also considered valid indications for subcision.(2, 10)

Advantages/disadvantages

The main advantage of subcision is that it has the potential to produce long-term improvement in the appearance of rolling acne scars while causing minimal injury to overlying skin. The procedure is easy to perform and is generally safe and well tolerated. Although it causes some bruising and swelling, the recovery time for subcision is brief. In addition, the materials used during the procedure are both inexpensive and widely available.

One disadvantage of subcision is that a single treatment is not guaranteed to produce substantial improvement. Because the final result of the procedure depends on a patient's individual wound-healing response, it is often difficult to predict the outcome of an initial treatment.(2) In order to achieve optimal results, some patients require several treatment sessions or adjunct procedures such as resurfacing or fillers.(2)

Complications

Erythema, bruising, edema, and tenderness are expected sequelae and may persist at the subcision site for 1 to 2 weeks.(2, 11) One potential complication is the formation of cystic acneiform lesions, which are thought to result from disruption of acne sinus tracts or pilosebaceous units.(2, 11)

While partial improvement of a depressed scar is common, an excessive or hypertrophic response may also occur in 5% to 10% of cases.(2, 11) An excessive response usually results in a small, palpable induration at the treated site.(12) Such areas of firmness may not be visible and may typically flatten over time. Patients may be informed that palpable but invisible bumps may be desirable to the extent that they tend to improve the smoothness of the final skin contour.

Combination Possibilities

Subcision may be readily combined with other procedures such as fillers (13), and nonablative (14) and ablative laser resurfacing.(15) In many instances, a combined treatment protocol will produce superior results, especially when rolling scars are interspersed with other forms of acne scars.

Practical advice for the clinician

Some bleeding and ecchymosis during the procedure is considered normal and beneficial, as it is thought that the collection of blood beneath the defect may instigate new collagen formation.(11) (Figure 12.1)

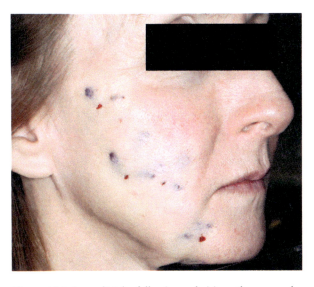

Figure 12.1 Immediately following subcision, there may be bleeding and ecchymosis at the treated sites. This is expected, and it may be beneficial in promoting the formation of new collagen beneath the depressed scars.

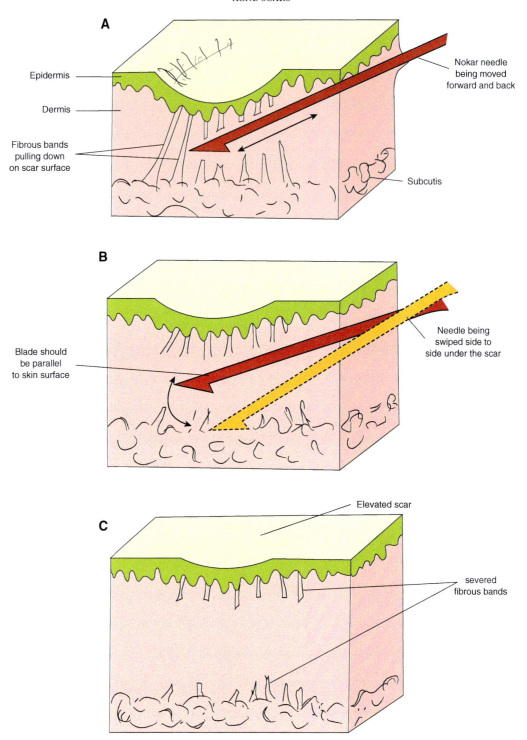

Figure 12.2 Subcision. (A) A NoKor needle (Becton Dickinson, Franklin Lakes, NJ, USA) is inserted at an angle into the skin adjacent to the scar so that its blade lies directly beneath the depressed area and is parallel to the skin surface. The needle is first advanced in a back-and-forth tunneling motion to pierce through the fibrous tissue. (B) Next, the needle is swept from side to side beneath the scar to ensure that all tethers are cut. (C) After healing, the scar is no longer bound down to the subcutis and its surface has elevated.

Prior to treatment, it is important for patients to understand that complete improvement after a single treatment with subcision is unlikely and several sessions may be required to achieve maximal correction.

Technical procedure

Before beginning the procedure, the skin is cleansed and the depressed scars are carefully outlined using a surgical marking pen. These sites are then infiltrated with a solution of 1% lidocaine with 1:100,000 epinephrine. The anesthetized area should extend far enough beyond the borders of each scar to allow for painless needle insertion. Once adequate anesthesia and vasoconstriction is achieved, a tribevelled hypodermic needle (2) or NoKor needle (11, 12) (Becton Dickinson, Franklin Lakes, NJ, USA) is inserted into the skin adjacent to the depression and advanced at an angle until it lies directly beneath the scar. (Figure 12.2) The depth of needle insertion will depend upon the severity of each scar, with more superficial scars being subcised at the level of the mid-dermis, and more deeply depressed scars being undermined in the deep dermis or subcutis.(11)

Initially, the subcision needle is moved forwards and backwards in a tunneling motion to pierce through the tough, fibrotic scar tissue. (Figure 12.2) Once the fibrous mass is sufficiently fragmented, the needle is swiped side to side in a direction parallel to the skin surface to free the scar from its tethers. (Figure 12.2) For densely fibrous scars, it may be useful to use several needle insertion sites to undermine the defect from different angles.(1) Upon severing the final tethers, the skin may visibly elevate.

Following the procedure, antibiotic ointment and a compression bandage may be applied.(1)

Management of Complications

If a cyst forms at a subcision site, it may be treated with intralesional steroid injection and oral antibiotics.

Indurations caused by hypertrophic response will usually disappear without intervention, but their resolution may be accelerated by daily firm fingertip massage of the sites (12) or low-dose intralesional corticosteroid injections.(1, 2, 11)

DERMAL GRAFTING

History

Dermal grafts and dermal-fat grafts have been used since the 1930's(16), but they were initially employed primarily for the correction of defects in organs other than the skin.(7, 17, 18) For many decades, the use of dermal grafts was limited by their tendency toward cyst formation and inconsistent results.(17, 18) However, recent improvements in harvesting and graft placement techniques have allowed dermal grafting to gain acceptance as an option for permanent augmentation of cutaneous depressions.(18)

Structure and Function

In the dermal grafting procedure, a depressed recipient site is undermined immediately prior to implantation of the graft. This step is designed to create a recipient pocket lined with highly vascular granulation tissue that can accept the graft and promote anastomosis of capillaries.(17) It is thought that this encourages rapid restoration of circulation to the graft and is consequently responsible for the high success rate of the procedure.(17)

Technology

Indication

Dermal grafting is indicated for the correction of broad (3 mm–2 cm in diameter) and linear scars that are soft and distensible.(17, 19) Like subcision, dermal grafting can augment depressed scars while leaving the overlying epidermis largely intact, so it is best suited to treat scars with normal overlying skin and a lack of sharp walls. Dermal grafting has also been used to augment wider, deep rhytids such as nasolabial folds and glabellar creases (17) and to correct deep nasal and alar rim defects resulting from Mohs surgery.(20)

Advantages and disadvantages

Dermal grafting is a useful technique for correcting deep contour defects and the grafts have several advantages over other augmenting agents. They are readily available, inexpensive, autologous implants that are nonallergenic and not susceptible to rejection.(7, 18) They also have the potential to provide long-term or permanent correction.(18) Furthermore, the grafts can be precisely altered to match the size and shape of nearly any depressed area.(7) Like subcision, dermal grafting spares a scar's surface from injury and typically results in only mild bruising and swelling.

The primary disadvantage of dermal grafting is that it requires a donor site, and patients and physicians may be reluctant to create a new defect. In addition, although dermal grafts have some advantages over other fillers, the process of harvesting and implanting the grafts is considerably more time consuming and challenging than alternative augmenting procedures. The increasing availability of numerous safe and relatively long-acting prepackaged injectable soft-tissue augmentation materials has resulted in a reduced interest in dermal grafting.

Complications

Following dermal grafting, some bruising, edema, and crusting at the insertion sites are expected.(7) The most frequent complication is cyst formation, which has an incidence of approximately 10%.(20) The best way to avoid this outcome is to take meticulous care to completely remove the epidermis and appendageal structures from the donor sites before harvesting grafts.(18)

Combination possibilities

Multiple dermal grafts may be implanted at different sites during the same procedure, which is advantageous in that it allows a single donor site to be used. In addition, dermal grafting may be performed at the same time as resurfacing.(18)

Practical advice for the clinician

Although dermal grafting is recommended for the treatment of distensible scars, one or two sessions of subcision may make some fibrotic scars soft enough to accept dermal grafting.(18)

When selecting punches to harvest round dermal grafts, it should be noted that while epidermal punch grafts are normally designed to be slightly larger than their recipient sites to allow for graft shrinkage, a dermal punch graft should exactly match the size and shape of the recipient defect.(18)

Technical Procedure

There is some difference of opinion concerning the optimal preparation for dermal grafting. While Swinehart recommends undermining a scar 10 to 14 days prior to graft placement and then again at the time of the procedure, (21) others prefer to subcise the scar only at the time of dermal grafting.(18) Regardless of whether this additional step is taken, immediately prior to dermal grafting, scars should be examined carefully in overhead or tangential light and both the scars and donor site should be carefully outlined with a marking pen. Photographs should be taken both before and after marking, and the postmarking photographs should be available as a reference during the procedure.

Next, both the donor and recipient sites are injected with local anesthetic, usually 1% to 2% lidocaine with 1:100,000 epinephrine, to achieve anesthesia and hemostasis. The donor site, which is typically the postauricular crease, is then deepithelialized to a level below the papillary dermis using either dermabrasion (7) or resurfacing laser.(19) Care should be taken to remove all appendageal structures, especially sebaceous glands that may lead to cyst formation if left behind.(18) Once the donor site is sufficiently deepithelialized, the method of graft harvesting will depend on the size and shape of the defect to be corrected. A scalpel or laser may be used to remove linear strips of dermis, while appropriately sized punches are ideal for producing grafts destined for small, round scars. The grafts should be placed in chilled sterile saline and, if necessary, they should be precisely trimmed to fit the recipient scar sites.(17)

Before implanting the graft, the scar should be freshly undermined to create a pocket underneath its depressed surface. For smaller, round scars, grafts may be inserted into their recipient pockets through the opening made by the subcision needle and manipulated into place with diamond-tipped jeweler's forceps.(17) (Figure 12.3)

For the correction of a larger linear scar, Goodman suggests using an intravenous cannula both to undermine the scar and to provide a means of guiding the graft into place.(18) The cannula is inserted at the one end of the linear defect, and after it is passed forward and backward several times to create the recipient pocket, it is passed out via the distal end of the scar.(18) Then, the plastic sleeve surrounding the instrument is left behind as the introducer is removed so that the sleeve protrudes from both ends of the recipient pocket.(19) This sleeve acts as a tunnel into which one can pull a dermal graft attached with a PDS suture to a straight needle.(18) The needle is passed through the distal end of the

tunnel until the graft is about to enter the sleeve, then the trailing end of the graft is grasped with jeweler's forceps so that it can be more easily manipulated into its final position.(18) With the graft still held by the jeweler's forceps, the sleeve and graft are pulled through the recipient tunnel as a unit so that the plastic sleeve is removed, and only the graft remains in the tunnel.(18) Once the graft is in a satisfactory position, the jeweler's forceps are removed and the suture is cut proximally.(18) Removal of the suture from the graft is not required. If necessary, the ends of the graft may be secured in place with highly degradable sutures and the ends of the recipient tunnel may be closed with Steri-strips (3M Corp, St. Paul, MN) or fine degradable sutures.(17) Finally, the donor site should be closed using a horizontal running mattress suture.(18)

Following the procedure, the patient should be advised to immobilize the graft site as much as possible for one to two days in order to maximize graft survival.(18) Immediate results of dermal grafting are typically very good, with complete or nearly complete correction of the defect evident upon dressing removal.(17) Unfortunately, these impressive initial results may not be permanent, as some grafts tend to lose volume over time. Nonetheless, in Goodman's 1997 study involving 11 patients with 32 dermal grafts, 84% of the grafts provided substantial improvement or complete correction of defects at follow-up periods from 3 to 30 months.(19)

Management of Complications

In the event of cyst formation, intralesional corticosteroid injections may be used. Alternatively, cysts may be drained or excised.(17)

EXCISION, PUNCH ELEVATION, AND PUNCH GRAFTING

History

Excision and punch techniques have been used for the past several decades in the revision of deep, atrophic acne scars.(8, 22–26) Today, these techniques remain indispensable for the correction of acne scars whose depth precludes correction by resurfacing and whose irregular scar bases and sharply defined walls make them unsuitable candidates for fillers.

Technology

Indication

Elliptical or punch excision should be used when one's aesthetic goal is to replace a prominent scar with a less conspicuous linear, superficial scar. Punch excision is indicated for the treatment of ice-pick and deep boxcar scars that are <3.5 mm in diameter.(1) Scars larger than 3.5 mm should be repaired with elliptical excision so that the resultant wound can be closed more effectively without the risk of "dog-ear" formation. Excision is also often the best option for the treatment of acne scars with cutaneous bridges or persistent cysts and tunnels.(27) It may also be an option for certain hypertrophic or keloidal acne scars.(21) (Table 12.2)

For some patients with icepick and deep boxcar scars, punch grafting may produce better cosmetic results than excision,

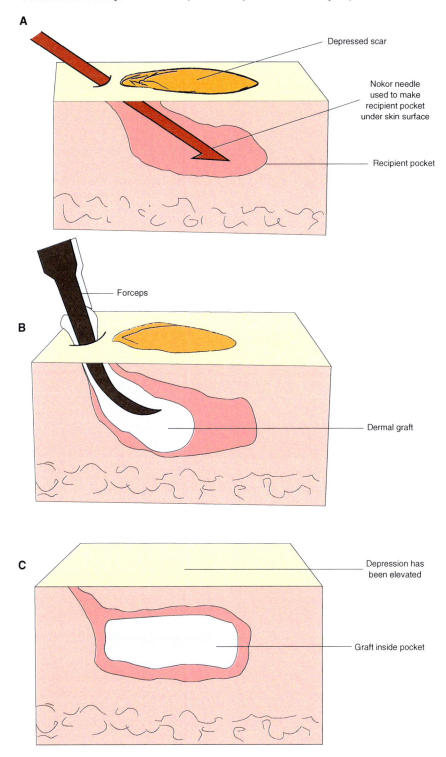

Figure 12.3 Dermal grafting. (A) The depressed scar is first subcised to create a recipient pocket for the graft. (B) Using jeweler's forceps, a freshly harvested dermal graft is inserted into the recipient pocket through the incision made by the subcision needle. (C) Upon completion of the procedure, the depressed area is augmented to the level of the surrounding skin.

Table 12.2 Indications for excision and punch techniques.

Technique	Indicated Scar Types
Punch excision	Ice-pick scars; deep boxcar scars <3.5 mm in diameter
Elliptical excision	Ice-pick scars; deep boxcar scars ≥3.5 mm in diameter; scars with bridges, cysts, or tunnels
Punch grafting	Ice-pick scars; deep boxcars scars
Punch elevation	Deep boxcar scars with vertical walls and scar bases that match surrounding skin in texture and pigmentation

particularly if the scars are in regions of the face where linear defects are not easily hidden in relaxed skin-tension lines. However, punch grafting is only feasible if the patient has a suitable donor site with skin that matches the scar site in color and texture. In addition, punch grafting is most successful in less mobile areas of the face such as the forehead and upper cheeks.(21) (Table 12.2)

Punch elevation has a very narrow indication for deep boxcar scars with bases that are smoothly textured, normal in pigmentation, and not fibrotic. The scars must also have vertical walls, as a scar that tapers along its depth would not have a large enough base to fill its surface opening. (Table 12.2)

Advantages and Disadvantages

Excision and punch techniques have a distinct advantage over nonsurgical scar revision techniques in their capacity to substantially improve the appearance of ice-pick and deep boxcar scarring. Until the recent development of the focal trichloroacetic acid technique (CROSS) for the treatment of narrow ice-pick scars, (28) cold-steel surgical techniques were the only effective treatments for deep, sharply punched-out acne scars and scars with irregular atrophic bases.

The primary disadvantage of all excision and punch techniques is that they necessitate the creation of secondary defects. The concept of replacing old scars with fresh ones may be unappealing to some patients and physicians. In addition, these procedures are unlikely to produce optimal results in patients with tendencies toward poor wound healing. It should be noted that some patients develop severe acne scars due to a propensity toward abnormal healing, and these particular patients would be poor candidates for these interventions. Even when performed in well-selected candidates, excision and punch techniques carry the risk of leaving behind conspicuously elevated or depressed scars. Punch grafting has the added disadvantages of requiring a donor site and involving the risks of graft extrusion or visual mismatch between the graft and recipient skin.

Complications

Following elliptical excision, depression and widening of scars may occur, particularly in regions of high sebaceous gland activity.(29, 30) This outcome is best prevented by careful patient selection and meticulous technique. While excising the defect, care should be taken to preserve as much subcutaneous tissue as possible to act as an anchoring foundation for the healing wound.(29) Precise suturing technique (31) and use of Steri-strips (3M Corp., St. Paul, MN) for up to 10 days following the procedure (32) can prevent scar spread. In addition, when planning to treat more substantial areas of scarring, large excisions should be avoided in favor of a series of small excisions performed at 4 to 6 week intervals.(31)

Some complications of punch transplantation include poor graft take, graft extrusion, depressed grooves around the margins of the grafts, depressed or elevated grafts, and color or texture mismatch between grafts and surrounding skin. To prevent these outcomes, the donor site should be carefully selected prior to the procedure. The risk of depressed borders around the grafts or depression or elevation of the grafts themselves can be minimized by ensuring that the graft is slightly larger in diameter than the recipient site and using Steri-strips(3M Corp., St. Paul, MN) to hold the grafts in place for a minimum of 5 days. (33) To decrease the chance of graft extrusion, patients should be advised not to touch or press on their graft sites and to minimize their facial movements for the 3 days following the surgery. (33) In addition, grafts are less likely to take in the lower cheeks and perioral area due to mouth and jaw movement. If grafts are placed in these areas, extra care should be taken to secure them in place, and patients should be strongly advised to limit talking and chewing for several days following the procedure.(33)

In punch elevation, the most frequent complication is persistent elevation of a plug above the level of the surrounding skin.(33)

Combination Possibilities

Excision and punch techniques are frequently combined with resurfacing procedures in order to improve the appearance of secondary defects. Traditionally, dermabrasion would be performed 4 to 8 weeks after excision or punch grafting; (23) however, a newer alternative is to perform a single combined procedure of laser resurfacing and excision or punch grafting.(34, 35)

Practical advice for the clinician

Because these procedures involve the creation of secondary defects, it is essential that patients have realistic expectations prior to undergoing excision or punch procedures. Patients should be well informed about the potential outcomes, and they should be willing to accept the possibility that subsequent procedures, such as laser resurfacing, may be necessary to produce an optimal result.

With all of these techniques, it is possible to treat multiple areas simultaneously. If two or more scars are to be excised, they should be at least 4 to 5 mm apart to prevent excess traction during healing.(1) If multiple punch transplants of different sizes are to be performed in a single procedure, it is helpful to devise a way of organizing and labeling the grafts before starting.

In punch grafting, careful donor-site selection is crucial. The postauricular area is most frequently used, but if it is not a good match with the recipient site or if it has active acne lesions, other sites, including the preauricular area, supraclavicular area, backs of the arms, and hairline, may be considered.(33)

Technical Procedure

Prior to an excision or punch procedure, scars are examined and marked, the area to be treated is properly cleansed, and the tissue is infiltrated with 1% lidocaine plus epinephrine (1:100,000.) For all punch techniques, a variety of disposable punch biopsy instruments are available, with diameters ranging in 0.25mm increments from 1.5 mm to 3.5 mm. (Goodman GJ, unpublished work) The walls of the punches are seamless and straight.

For punch excision, a punch instrument is selected that is just large enough to encompass the scar, including its walls. (1) The first finger and thumb are placed on either side of the scar and used to create outward traction perpendicular to a resting skin tension line.(21) This will result in an elongated wound that will be camouflaged along a natural facial line. The punch is inserted at a 90-degree angle and inserted to the level of the subcutaneous fat; unless the scar's base is very fibrotic, it will easily lift out. If necessary, forceps and iris scissors can be used to gently release the scar from any fibrous attachments. (1) If smaller than 2 mm, a wound may be left to heal by second intention (30) or it may be closed with one or two simple, interrupted sutures.(1) Punch sites larger than 2.5 mm may heal better when closed with a single buried-deep suture.(1) If sutures are used, they are removed within 7 days to prevent track-mark formation.(1)

For acne scars larger than 3 mm, elliptical excision is preferable to punch excision. A scalpel blade is used to excise an ellipse oriented longitudinally along a resting skin tension line. The scar is encompassed at the center of the ellipse and the wound angles are 30 degrees or less to allow for aesthetic closure.(21) Undermining may be used to mobilize the wound edges for tension-free wound closure.(32) Small excisions may be closed with buried dermal sutures (31) while larger excisions may be closed with several simple, interrupted sutures (1) or buried vertical mattress (21) sutures.

To perform punch elevation, a punch instrument is chosen that exactly matches the diameter of the scar base. (Figure 12.4) The punch is inserted down to the level of subcutaneous fat so that the tissue may be manipulated.(33) Next, forceps are used to gently elevate the scar base until it sits slightly higher than the surrounding surface, and the tissue is held in place for 1 or 2 minutes until a coagulum forms beneath it.(33) (Figure 12.4) The plug is then secured in place using sutures, Dermabond (2-Octyl Cyanoacrylate, Ethicon, Inc., Somerville, NJ), or Steri-strips (3M Corp., St. Paul, MN).(21) The area is covered with bacitracin and dressed with gauze, and the patient is instructed to gently wash the area and reapply bacitracin twice a day.(1)

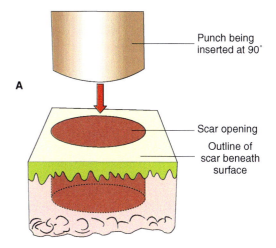

Punch being inserted at 90°

Scar opening

Outline of scar beneath surface

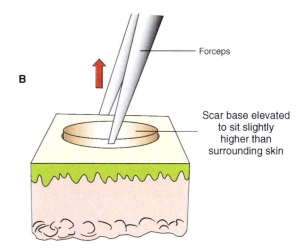

Forceps

Scar base elevated to sit slightly higher than surrounding skin

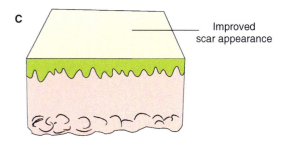

Improved scar appearance

Figure 12.4 Punch elevation of a deep boxcar scar. (A) A punch is selected that matches the diameter of the scar base and is inserted at a 90° angle down to the level of the subcutaneous tissue. (B) Forceps are then used to gently elevate the scar base so that it sits slightly higher than the surrounding skin. (C) The elevated plug should flatten on its own during healing.

Prior to punch grafting, an appropriate donor site is pre-pared and anesthetized in the same manner as recipient site. First, the entire scar, including its walls, is excised. (Figure 12.5) The punch should be inserted at a 90-degree angle to the skin surface with a twisting motion. In contrast with the punch excision procedure described above, care should be taken to avoid lateral stretching of the skin so that the resulting recipient hole will be perfectly round.(27) The excised scars are removed and discarded. A graft is then harvested using a punch 0.25 to 0.5 mm larger in diameter using the same proce-dure to create a full-thickness, cylindrical graft. Use of a slightly larger graft is recommended because grafts have a tendency to contract while the recipient wounds may expand, and it is important for the graft to maintain contact with the margins of the recipient hole.(23, 27) Using forceps, the graft is gen-tly inserted and manipulated into the recipient site so that its surface rests slightly higher than the surrounding skin.(Figure 12.5) Finally, the graft is either sutured or glued in place and secured with Steri-strips (3M Corp., St. Paul, MN), and the donor site is sutured closed. Patients should be advised to limit their facial movements and to avoid touching graft sites for the first several days.

Management of Complications

As described above, the risk of complications from excision and punch procedures may be minimized through careful technique. With larger punch excisions and elliptical exci-sions, meticulous suturing is necessary to produce the least conspicuous secondary defects. In punch grafting, careful donor-site selection, precise harvesting techniques, and pains-taking graft placement are all integral to the achievement of a good result.

When secondary defects are not aesthetically acceptable, their appearance can often be improved with subsequent procedures. An elevated graft or plug or raised excision scar is often ade-quately managed by laser resurfacing performed approximately 4 to 8 weeks after the original procedure.(25) In the event of punch graft extrusion or the development of a depressed scar, the original procedure should be repeated.(23, 27)

In punch elevation, plugs that are initially elevated above the level of the surrounding skin usually flatten without interven-tion, but persistently elevated plugs may be planed with resur-facing performed at 4 to 8 weeks after the original procedure. (Goodman GJ, unpublished work)

OUTLOOK—FUTURE DEVELOPMENTS

While many of the surgical treatments for acne scarring have been in use for decades, there has been a very limited amount of research evaluating the long-term response to these treatments and comparing outcomes from different treatments. Such work might lead to improved outcomes by refining surgical tech-niques and altering treatment protocols.

Recent work in stem-cell biology and regenerative medicine suggests that novel approaches to scar revision may be available

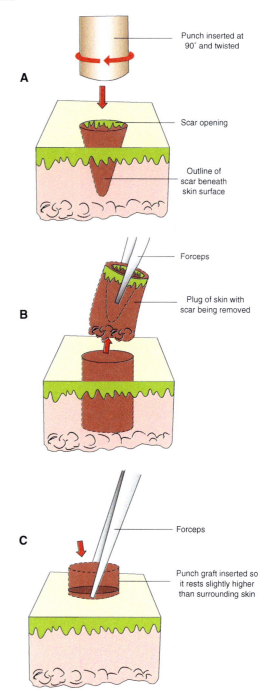

Figure 12.5 Punch grafting of an ice-pick scar. (A) A punch is selected that will fully encompass the scar and its walls and is inserted at a 90° with a twisting motion down to the level of the subcutis. (B) Next, forceps are used to remove the scar from the recipient hole. (C) A full-thickness graft that is slightly larger than the recipient hole is inserted using forceps. Its surface should rest slightly higher than the surrounding skin.

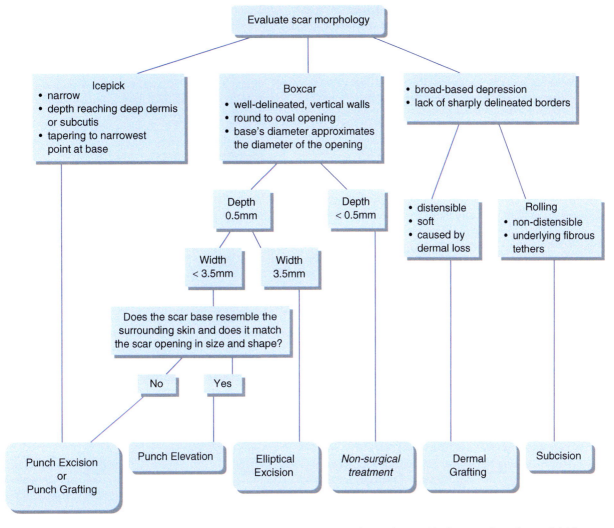

Figure 12.6 Flowchart linking different acne scar types to appropriate surgical procedures. With the exception of superficial boxcar scars <0.5 mm in depth, each scar type may be improved by surgical revision. Punch excision and punch grafting are suitable for treating ice-pick and deep boxcar scars, punch elevation may be used to correct deep boxcar scars with regular bases, subcision is ideal for treating rolling scars, and dermal grafting is an option for improving distensible depressed scars.

in the future. Great strides have been made in elucidating the differences between the process of fibrotic wound healing that leads to scarring and the pathways that produce perfect regeneration of injured tissues, a phenomenon that can be observed in human fetuses and other organisms.(36) Skin progenitor cells have already been identified in mammals, and it is expected that by grafting such cells into injured skin and providing the right microenvironmental conditions, healing by regeneration may be induced.(36) Thus, it may eventually become possible to excise a fibrotic scar and manipulate the resultant wound in such a way that it will be replaced by normal, healthy skin.

SUMMARY FOR THE CLINICIAN
Revision of acne scarring is a complex task in which treatment protocols are designed on a case-by-case basis following critical evaluation of scars and thorough consideration of patients' preferences and goals. As each scar revision technique is best suited to address a subset of scars, being equipped to treat the full range of acne scarring requires familiarizing oneself with a variety of procedures. The surgical techniques described in this chapter are essential components of such a repertoire, and they are among the few procedures capable of improving deep and fibrotic acne scars.(Figure 12.6) Because severe acne scars are

frequently the source of profound social and emotional distress for patients, learning these techniques will be worthwhile for the cosmetic dermatologist.

REFERENCES

1. Jacob CI, Dover JS, Kaminer MS. Acne scarring: a classification system and review of treatment options. J Am Acad Dermatol 2001; 45: 109–17.
2. Orentreich DS, Orentreich N. Subcutaneous incisionless (subcision) surgery for the correction of depressed scars and wrinkles. Dermatol Surg 1995; 21: 543–9.
3. Spangler AS. New treatment for pitted scars; preliminary report. AMA Arch Derm 1957; 76: 708–11.
4. Treatment of depressed cutaneous scars with gelatin matrix implant: a multicenter study. J Am Acad Dermatol 1987; 16: 1155–62.
5. Cohen I. Fibrel®. Semin Dermatol 1987; 6: 228–37.
6. Hambley RM, Carruthers JA. Microlipoinjection for the elevation of depressed full-thickness skin grafts on the nose. J Dermatol Surg Oncol 1992; 18: 963–8.
7. Swinehart J. Pocket grafting with dermal grafts: autologous collagen implants for permanent correction of cutaneous depressions. Amer J Cosm Surg 1995; 12: 321–31.
8. Orentreich D, Orentreich N. Acne scar revision update. Dermatol Clin 1987; 5: 359–68.
9. Goodman GJ. Post-acne scarring: a short review of its pathophysiology. Australas J Dermatol 2001; 42: 84–90.
10. Hexsel DM, Mazzuco R. Subcision: a treatment for cellulite. Int J Dermatol 2000; 39: 539–44.
11. Goodman GJ. Therapeutic undermining of scars (Subcision). Australas J Dermatol 2001; 42: 114–7.
12. Alam M, Omura N, Kaminer MS. Subcision for acne scarring: technique and outcomes in 40 patients. Dermatol Surg 2005; 31: 310–7.
13. Balighi K, Robati RM, Moslehi H, Robati AM. Subcision in acne scar with and without subdermal implant: a clinical trial. J Eur Acad Dermatol Venereol 2008; 22: 707–11.
14. Fulchiero GJ Jr, Parham-Vetter PC, Obagi S. Subcision and 1320 nm Nd:YAG nonablative laser resurfacing for the treatment of acne scars: a simultaneous split-face single patient trial. Dermatol Surg 2004; 30: 1356–9.
15. Branson DF. Dermal undermining (scarification) of active rhytids and scars: enhancing the results of CO2 laser skin resurfacing. Aesthet Surg J 1998; 18: 36–7.
16. Peer LA, Paddock R. Histologic studies on the fate of deeply implanted dermal grafts: observations on secions of implants buried from one week to one year. Arch Surg 1937; 34: 268.
17. Swinehart JM. Dermal grafting. Dermatol Clin 2001; 19: 509–22.
18. Goodman GJ. Autologous fat and dermal grafting for the correction of facial scars. In: Surgical Techniques for Cutaneous Scar Revsion. Harahap M, ed. New York: Marcel Dekker, 2000: 311–48.
19. Goodman G. Laser-assisted dermal grafting for the correction of cutaneous contour defects. Dermatol Surg 1997; 23: 95–9.
20. Meyers S, Rohrer T, Grande D. Use of dermal grafts in reconstructing deep nasal defects and shaping the ala nasi. Dermatol Surg 2001; 27: 300–5.
21. Choi JM, Rohrer TE, Kaminer MS, Batra RS. Surgical Approaches to Patients with Scarring. In: Scar Revision. Arndt KA, ed. Elsevier Saunders, 2006: 45–66.
22. Solotoff SA. Treatment for pitted acne scarring–postauricular punch grafts followed by dermabrasion. J Dermatol Surg Oncol 1986; 12: 1079–84.
23. Johnson WC. Treatment of pitted scars: punch transplant technique. J Dermatol Surg Oncol 1986; 12: 260–5.
24. Stal S, Hamilton S, Spira M. Surgical treatment of acne scars. Clin Plast Surg 1987; 14: 261–76.
25. Dzubow LM. Scar revision by punch-graft transplants. J Dermatol Surg Oncol 1985; 11: 1200–2.
26. Eiseman G. Reconstruction of the acne-scarred face. J Dermatol Surg Oncol 1977; 3: 332–8.
27. Stegman SJ. Cosmetic Dermatologic Surgery. 2nd ed. Chicago: Year Book Medical Publishers, Inc. 1990.
28. Lee JB, Chung WG, Kwahck H, Lee KH. Focal treatment of acne scars with trichloroacetic acid: chemical reconstruction of skin scars method. Dermatol Surg 2002; 28: 1017–21.
29. Tsao SS, Dover JS, Arndt KA, Kaminer MS. Scar management: keloid, hypertrophic, atrophic, and acne scars. Semin Cutan Med Surg 2002; 21: 46–75.
30. Koranda FC. Treatment and modalities in facial acne scars. In: Facial Scars: Incision, Revision, and Camouflage. Thomas JR, Holt GR, eds. St. Louis: The C.V. Mosby Company, 1989: 278–89.
31. Haneke E. Fusiform Excision and Serial Excisions. In: Surgical Techniques for Cutaneous Scar Revsion. Harahap M, ed. New York: Marcel Dekker, 2000: 359–80.
32. Usatine R. Elliptical Excision. In: Skin Surgery: A Practical Guide. Usatine RP, Moy RL, eds. St. Louis: Mosby; 1998.
33. Griffin E. Punch Transplant Technique for Pitted Scars. In: Surgical Techniques for Cutaneous Scar Revision. Harahap M, ed. New York: Marcel Dekker, 2000: 259–74.
34. Grevelink JM, White VR. Concurrent use of laser skin resurfacing and punch excision in the treatment of facial acne scarring. Dermatol Surg 1998; 24: 527–30.
35. Goodman GJ. The limitations of skin resurfacing techniques. The necessity to combine procedures. Dermatol Surg 1998; 24: 687–8.
36. Gurtner GC, Werner S, Barrandon Y, Longaker MT. Wound repair and regeneration. Nature 2008; 453: 314–21.

13 Camouflage: Clinical importance of corrective cover cosmetic (Camouflage) and quality-of-life outcome in the management of patients with acne scarring and/or post-inflammatory hyperpigmentation

Aurora Tedeschi and Lee E West

INTRODUCTION

Dermatologic disorders can be very distressing to patients, especially when they are located in highly visible anatomic areas. Patients react negatively to the lack of eye contact when interacting with others; moreover, psychological effects of skin disorders include problems such as depression, loss of self-esteem, quality-of-life deterioration, sexual dysfunction, and increased prevalence of emotional distress as compared to the general population.(1–3) Some dermatologic conditions, such as acne, may result in scarring with varying degrees of cosmetic disfigurement despite a positive response to treatment or surgical management of the underlying inflammatory acne disorder.(4, 5)

Unfortunately, there are relatively few treatment options for acne scarring. Long-term therapy with topical retinoids may provide minimal improvement for those with mild scarring.(6) Surgical and medical procedural approaches to acne scars, such as punch or elliptical excision or punch elevation or chemical peeling and dermabrasion, may provide effective treatment in the hands of experienced practitioners, but they do present risks while making a decision about which method to choose that eventually benefit the patient and the doctor.(6)

Camouflage, or corrective cover cosmetic (CCC), may be used as an alternative to medications, procedures, and surgery and is notably used as a temporary postprocedure cover for erythema resulting from dermabrasion or chemical peel and may be used as an adjunct in the pharmacotherapeutic management of a number of dermatoses (Table 13.1).(7–13) In addition, CCC has been used as a supplement to dermatological therapy in order to provide a more positive outcome for the patient than may be achieved by therapy alone.(14) Finally, CCC is reported to improve mental well-being, self-esteem, and social acceptance.(15)

MATERIALS AND METHODS

Independent CCC clinics in two academic clinic settings in the United States (Chicago) and Italy (Catania) pooled data on patients with acne scarring and/or postinflammatory hyperpigmentation who received CCC. Patients consulting the CCC clinics underwent a preliminary examination aimed to evaluate the need, expectations, and likely outcome for CCC, patient lifestyle, and to provide more detailed information about CCC. Quality of life (QoL) and the relationship between acne scarring and degree of psychological discomfort was also evaluated.(7–10)

Table 13.1 Selected dermatoses manageable with Corrective Cover Cosmetic.

Acne
Acne scars
Achanthosis nigricans
Allergic contact dermatitis
Becker nevus
Blue nevus
Burn scars
Chloasma/Melasma
Guttate idiopathic hypomelanosis
Lentigo
Lichen verrucosus
Melanocytic nevus
Nevus of Ota
Palpebral hyperpigmentation
Postinflammatory immunobullous disorders (i.e., pemphigus)
Psoriasis
Rosacea
Surgery scars
Telangiectasias
Xeroderma pigmentosum
Vitiligo

The CCC clinics stressed the importance of a private, screened area for patient consultation and CCC application to provide for confidentiality, as a safe, secluded environment for treatment is perceived to be as important as treatment itself by such patients.

CCC-eligible patients with acne scarring and/or postinflammatory hyperpigmentation routinely underwent education for skin cleansing and hydrating procedures with nonallergenic and noncomedogenic/nonacnegenic products. The most appropriate foundation color from a selection of light to very opaque, water-resistant or waterproof, noncomedogenic/nonacnegenic and/or hypoallergenic products was also applied and fixed with powder application.

Alterations in pigment were corrected through the application of green and/or yellow undercover, in order to respectively neutralize reddish and gray/brownish or blue defects; for postinflammatory hyperpigmentation, as may be commonly seen with facial acne, green undercover was commonly used as a masking technique.(7–10)

Patients returned to the CCC clinic 2 weeks later in order to reinforce education and technique as well as to obtain follow-up on QoL.

RESULTS

Over a 4-year period, in the dermatology departments of the University of Catania and of Northwestern University, between May 2001 and July 2005, 183 patients with facial acne scarring with or without postinflammatory hyperpigmentation received CCC. The most common disorder managed by CCC was acne scarring with or without postinflammatory hyperpigmentation. Selected examples of such patients who received CCC are shown in Figures 13.1–13.6.

Despite a less than optimal CCC outcome, overall, those with acne scarring and/or postinflammatory acne facial hyperpigmentation reported a higher degree of satisfaction with

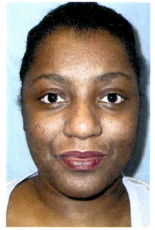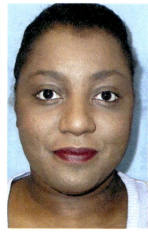

Figure 13.3 Scars on dark skin: before and after camouflage.

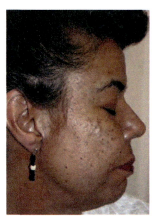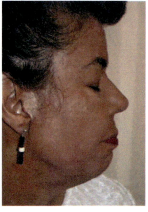

Figure 13.1 Scars and hyperpigmentation on dark skin before and after camouflage.

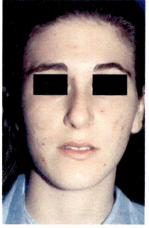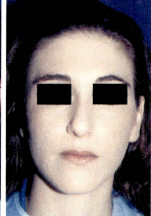

Figure 13.4 Patient with scars before and after camouflage.

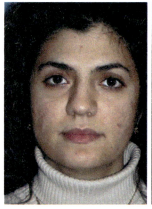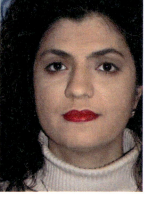

Figure 13.2 Deep scars before and after camouflage.

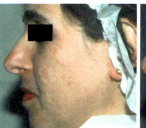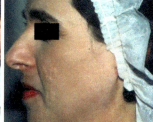

Figure 13.5 Postacneic scars and dyschromic lesions before and after camouflage.

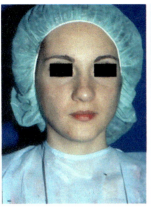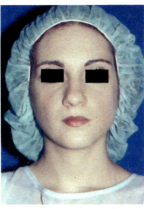

Figure 13.6 Papules and postinflammatory erythematous lesions before and after camouflage.

CCC than was reported with other, more easily camouflaged, dermatoses.

DISCUSSION

CCC is reported to have been introduced in the United States in the late 1960s (16, 17) and in France in the early 1980s. Subsequently, CCC use became even more widespread as reported for the United Kingdom and Italy.(18) CCC represents a noninvasive technique that may improve quality of life as a singular approach to a cosmetic dermatologic disorder or as an adjunct to treatment of various dermatoses. Patients can be easily educated to understand CCC, and the side effects associated with CCC are mostly mild and temporary, being limited to irritant or allergic contact dermatitis.

Notably, CCC now consists of technologically advanced formulations that may be noncomedogenic and nonacnegenic, but such formulations remain somewhat less successful in covering acne scars than for some other dermatologic disorders, which is primarily due to the difficulty in "filling" hypotrophic scars and the shadows formed by such scars (i.e., acne pitting) remain visible.

CONCLUSION

Two large academic-based CCC clinics pooled data to determine the utility, patient acceptance, and effect on QoL for patients with acne scarring and/or postinflammatory hyperpigmentation. CCC, in the hands of experienced practitioners, and provided in a private setting, proved to be well accepted, increased patient's quality of life, and served as a useful adjunct by providing complete or partial cover of cosmetic disfiguration in acne scarring and/or postinflammatory facial acne hyperpigmentation.

REFERENCES

1. Shuster S. Depression of self-image by skin disease. Acta Derm Venereol 1991; 156(Suppl): 53.
2. Kent G, Kehoane S. Social anxiety and disfigurement: the moderating effects of fear of negative evaluation and past experience. Br J Clin Psychol 2001; 40: 23–34.
3. Van Dorssen IE. Experience of sexuality in patients with psoriasis and constitutional eczema. Ned Tijdschr Geneeskd 1992; 136: 2175–8.
4. Graham JA, Jouhar AJ. The importance of cosmetics in the psychological of appearance. Int J Dermatol 1983; 22: 153–6.
5. Draelos ZD. Camouflaging techniques and dermatologic surgery. Dermatol Surg 1996; 22: 1023–7.
6. Rivera AE. Acne scarring: a review and current treatment modalities. J Am Acad Dermatol 2008; 59: 659–76.
7. Tedeschi A, Dall'Oglio F, Micali G, Schwartz RA, Janniger CK. Corrective camouflage in pediatric dermatology. Cutis 2007; 79: 110–2.
8. Tedeschi A, Dall'Oglio R, Micali G, Schwartz RA, Janniger CK. Corrective camouflage in dermatology practice. Aesthetic Dermatology 2003; 5: 273–5.
9. Tedeschi A, Dall'Oglio R, Micali G. Our experience in the corrective camouflage in dermatology practice. Proceedings 11th European Academy of Dermatology and Venerology (EADV) Congress, Prague, Czech Republic, October 2–6, 2002.
10. West LE, West D, Tedeschi A, Gallo E. A corrective cosmetic cover clinic within a dermatology practice. J Am Acad Dermatol 2004; 50(3 Suppl): P72.
11. Natow AJ. Corrective cosmetics. Cutis 1985; 36: 123–4.
12. Roberts NC. Corrective cosmetics – need, evaluation, and use. Cutis 1988; 41: 439–41.
13. Roberts FL, Forget BM. Application techniques for corrective and camouflage cosmetics. Ear Nose Throat J 1987; 66: 12–8.
14. Westmore MG. Make-up as an adjunct and aid to the practice of dermatology. Dermatol Clin 1991; 9: 81–8.
15. Grimes PE. Skin and hair cosmetic issues in women of color. Dermatol Clin 2000; 18: 659–65.
16. Cohen S. The use of "covermark" in the treatment of skin disfigurements. S Afr Med J 1965; 39: 301.
17. Jung HD. The treatment of disfiguring skin changes using water resistant make-up covermark. Z Aut Geschlechtskr 1970; 45: 351–6.
18. Caputo R, Barbareschi M, Baggini G, Bovo D. The corrective make-up lab: the Italian experience. Poster, 60th Meeting of the American Academy of Dermatology, New Orleans (LA), February 22nd–27th 2002.

14 Acne scars in Asian patients

Evangeline B Handog, Ma Juliet E Macarayo, and Ma Teresita G Gabriel

KEY FEATURES

- Acne scars among Asian patients do not vary much from the classical clinical acne scars seen worldwide.
- Postinflammatory hyperpigmentation as sequela of acne is more disturbing among Asian patients.
- Acne scars cause much distress not only to the patient but to the family as well.
- Prevention of acne scars rests on early and adequate management of acne.

INTRODUCTION

Acne among Asians is commonplace. A vast majority of acne patients develop scars. It is important to consider both the severity and delay of adequate treatment as factors. Understanding acne scarring among Asians would necessitate knowledge of "brown" skin.

Racial classifications have been more or less arbitrary with Asian skin being categorized under "skin of color or pigmented skin." As Homo sapiens, we were previously divided into five subspecies or races, with Asians being the representative people of the Mongoloid race. With migration, intermarriages, and overseas job opportunities, Asians are now a heterogeneous group, not anymore confined to simply being the "brown race." Asians have become a mixture of different cultures: Spanish, Malay, Chinese, Japanese, and Indians. Rarely can we see pure-blooded Asians.

In the skin phototype (SPT) system developed by Fitzpatrick, skin of color was initially classified as skin type V. Due to greater color gradations, skin of color was further subdivided into skin types IV, V, and VI. Asians generally belong to SPT IV-V but in various studies by Asian dermatologists, they found that Asian skin types encompassed SPT II–V.(1, 2) With the limitation of this current classification system, Kawasa (1986) (3) and Verallo-Rowell (2001) (4) adapted modifications of the Fitzpatrick skin phototyping system to fit the Japanese and Filipino populations, respectively.

Asian skin tone may vary from the lightest to the darkest of brown shade and texture variation may be from smooth and fine to rough and thick.

EPIDEMIOLOGY

Acne among Asians

Although there are published surveys on the prevalence of acne vulgaris in people of skin color, there is paucity focusing on Asian skin. Goh and Akarapanth (1994) noted that among 74,589 Asians consulting a Singapore clinic, it was the second most common diagnosis, seen in 10.9% of the adult patient population and the eighth top diagnosis in a pediatric population, occurring in 3.1% of those screened.(5) In a more recent survey, Yeung et al (2002) reported a prevalence of 52.2% among 522 Hong Kong adolescents aged 15 to 25 years.(6) In 2002, Roa et al's questionnaire survey (2004) among 114 Filipino dermatologists revealed that 44% of the respondents were managing more than 50% acne cases in their daily practice.(unpublished). Among 32,312 new consults at the Research Institute for Tropical Medicine (RITM), Department of Health, Philippines, acne vulgaris was the top dermatologic diagnosis between 2004 and 2007.(RITM Census).

Acne management, though greatly improved with modernization of times, relies heavily on the patients' desire to seek treatment and capacity to afford it. Only 2.4% of the Hong Kong adolescents beset with acne sought medical consult even if they were much disturbed by the condition psychologically and physically. Self-medication was done by 41.5%.(6) In Venida et al's study on 174 Filipinos with acne vulgaris, aged 14 to 50 years, 52% had treatment, more than half of which were self-medications rather than dermatologist-prescribed medications [RTD, Acne Board of the Philippines, 2007]. Acne scarring is thus a threatening sequelae posing a problem to both patients and dermatologists.

Acne Scarring among Filipinos

Postacne scarring is a very distressing and difficult problem for physicians and patients alike. Sulzberger and Zaidems emphasized that "There is no single disease which causes more psychic trauma, more maladjustment between parent and children, more general insecurity and feelings of inferiority and greater sums of psychic suffering than does acne vulgaris"(7)

In a recently concluded survey by the authors (August–November 2008) that involved 269 Filipino dermatologists on Acne Scarring, the age group where scarring is most commonly seen is between 26 and 35 years; 78% of the patients have typical Filipino "brown" skin and would fall under Fitzpatrick SPT-IV. In the majority of the respondents, approximately 41% to 60% of all acne patients complained of scarring on initial consult. Hyperpigmented acne scars were the predominant type of scarring observed in 84%, followed by depressed scars (80%), atrophic scars (67%), hypertrophic scars (55%), and hypopigmented scars (29%). Fifty three percent of the patients with scarring seen in private clinics expressed concern and wanted their acne scars to be treated. As to the preference in treating acne scars, 89% of the respondents treated 90% of their patients with the combination of topical preparations and procedural management. Retinoids and alpha hydroxy acids, alone or in combination with depigmenting agents are widely prescribed by our dermatologists. The different office procedures performed by the majority of the respondents to improve acne scarring in our setting are as follows: chemical peeling (86%), microdermabrasion (65%), microneedling (52%), lasers/light (43%), and laserbrasion (23%). Subcision, tissue augmentation, mechanical dermabrasion are being done by a few. In a survey conducted by the Skin of Color Center at New York City, the presence of dark marks or the acne hyperpigmented macule (AHM) among Black, Hispanic, and Asian patients were reported at 65.3%, 52.7%, and 47.4%, respectively. There was also a high reported incidence of keloidal scarring as a sequela of acne, occurring in 54.1% of all patients.(8)

HISTORY
The vast array of treatment modalities for acne vulgaris available in Western countries have been accessible to the Asian population as well. Treatment is encouraged even at the earliest stages of mild acne vulgaris, the goal of which is to lessen if not halt the occurrence of acne sequelae. A consensus from the Global Alliance to Improve Outcomes in Acne on Acne Treatment

has been made available since 2003. The Acne Board of the Philippines came up with its treatment guidelines on acne vulgaris in 2005.(Figure 14.1)

PATHOGENESIS OF ACNE VULGARIS
The pathogenesis of acne vulgaris is universal and basically the same for all races, be it Asian or Caucasian. There are no comparative racial studies analyzing differences in pilosebaceous follicle hyperkeratinization. Facial bacterial colonization by P. acnes in black skin was greater compared with white skin, but there is no similar study involving Asian skin or "brown skin." Few studies on racial differences in sebaceous gland size and activity exist, with extremely small number of subjects and contradictory results. A study done by Abedeen et al (2000) revealed no statistical difference in the rate of sebum production among 20 Whites, 20 Blacks, and 20 Asians.(9)

CLINICAL FEATURES
Acne vulgaris is categorized based on disease severity.(Table 14.1) Scarring can be a complication of both noninflammatory and inflammatory acne.(10) This may be greatly influenced by delay in effective treatment and degree of severity of acne. Two recent classification systems of acne scarring are available. Roberts Scarring Scale (Table 14.2) appears to be simple and

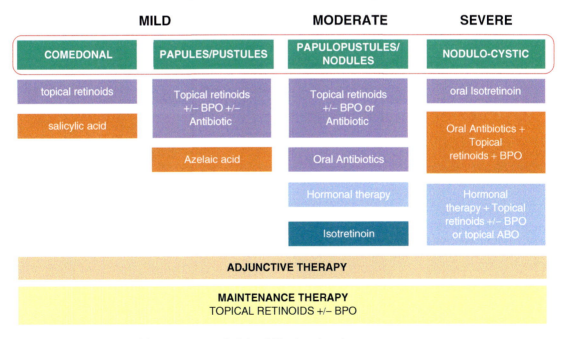

Figure 14.1 Acne Treatment Guidelines, Acne Board of the Philippines (2005).

easy to do. Goodman and Baron's Global Acne Scarring (Table 14.3) is more precise but very tedious to perform in a clinic set-up. In Southeast Asian countries, practicing clinicians will consider two important aspects of acne scarring: color and depth (Figure 14.2), with the former being the most troubling for the patient and the latter, for the dermatologist.

Postacne hyperpigmentary changes, although not true scars by definition, are commonly seen among Asians (Figure 14.3) This is postulated to be due to their higher epidermal melanin content.(11)

True acne scarring may be a result of either an excess or loss of tissue formation. Excess tissue formation is represented by hypertrophic scars and keloids, claimed to be 3 to 5x higher in Asians compared to Caucasians (12) (Figure 14.4) Loss of tissue, which is the more common sequela, is represented by the three primary acne scars (ice pick, box car, and rolling scars) and atrophic scars. (Figure 14.5, 14.6, 14.7, 14.8) Filipino dermatologists see more of the depressed compared to the elevated acne scars.

Table 14.1 Classification of Acne Severity.

Mild	Predominance of comedones ≤20 with few inflammatory papules ≤15
Moderate	Predominance of inflammatory papules and pustules ≥15 with comedones and few nodules ≤3
Severe	Primarily nodules and cysts ≥3 with presence of comedones, papules, and pustules

Source: Acne Board of the Philippines (2005).

Table 14.2 The Roberts Skin-Type Classification System.

Fitzpatrick (FZ) Scale: Measures skin phototypes

FZ 1	White skin; always burns, never tans
FZ 2	White skin; always burns, minimal tan
FZ 3	White skin; burns minimally, tans moderately and gradually
FZ 4	Light brown skin; burns minimally, tans well
FZ 5	Brown skin; rarely burns, tans deeply
FZ 6	Dark brown/black skin; never burns, tans deeply

Roberts Hyperpigmentation (H) Scale: propensity for pigmentation

H0	Hypopigmentation
H1	Minimal and transient (<1 year) hyperpigmentation
H2	Minimal and permanent (>1 year) hyperpigmentation
H3	Moderate and transient (<1 year) hyperpigmentation
H4	Moderate and permanent (>1 year) hyperpigmentation
H5	Severe and transient (<1 year) hyperpigmentation
H6	Severe and permanent (>1 year) hyperpigmentation

Glogau (G) Scale: describes photoaging

G1	No wrinkles, early photoaging
G2	Wrinkles in motion, early-to-moderate photoaging
G3	Wrinkles at rest, advanced photoaging
G4	Only wrinkles, severe photoaging

Roberts Scarring (S) Scale: describes scar morphology

S0	Atrophy
S1	None
S2	Macule
S3	Plaque within scar boundaries
S4	Keloid
S5	Keloidal nodule

Source: Four elements of the Roberts Skin Classification System.

Table 14.3 The Global Acne Scarring Classification System.

(Grade) Type	Number of Lesions: 1 (1–10)	Number of Lesions: 2 (11–20)	Number of Lesions: 3 (>20)
(A) Milder scarring (1 point each) Macular erythematous or pigmented Mildly atrophic dish like	1 point	2 points	3 points
(B) Moderate Scarring (2 points each) Moderately atrophic dish-like Punched out with shallow bases, small scars (<5 mm) Shallow but broad atrophic areas	2 points	4 points	6 points
(C) Severe Scarring (3 points each) Punched out with deep but normal bases, small scars (<5 mm) Punched out with deep abnormal bases, small scars (<5 mm) Linear or troughed dermal scarring Deep, broad atrophic areas	3 points	6 points	9 points
(D) Hyperplastic papular scars Hyperplastic Keloidal/hypertrophic scars	2 points Area < 5 cm^2 6 points	4 points Area 5 to 20 cm^2 12 points	6 points Area > 20 cm^2 18 points

Source: Goodman and Baron.

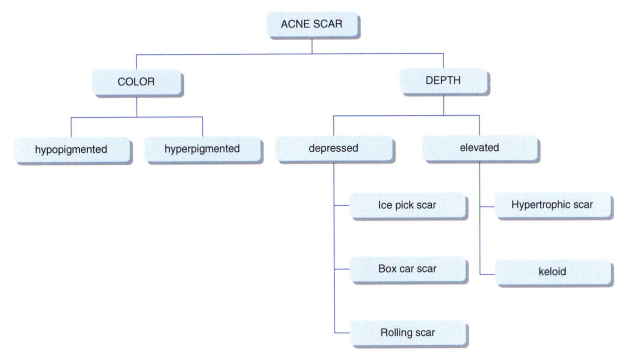

Figure 14.2 Acne Scar Classification by Color and Depth.

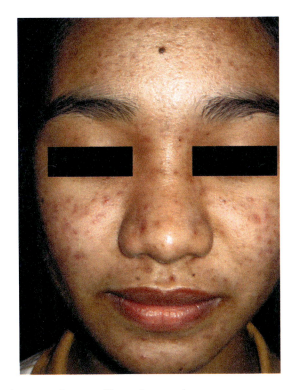

Figure 14.3 Postacne Hyperpigmentation.

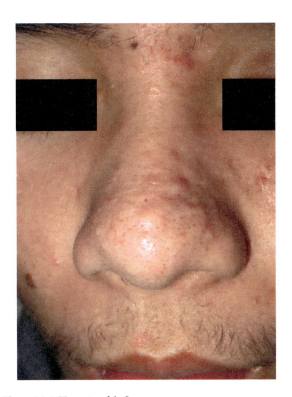

Figure 14.4 Hypertrophic Scars.

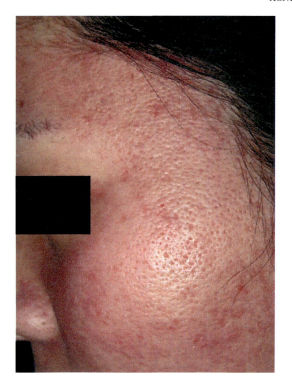

Figure 14.5 Ice-pick Scars.

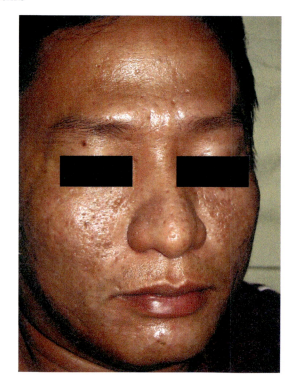

Figure 14.6 Boxcar Scars.

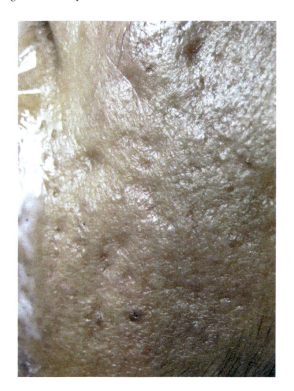

Figure 14.7 Rolling Scars.

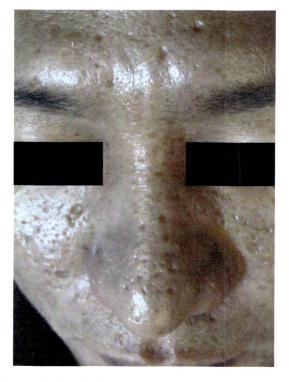

Figure 14.8 Atrophic Scars.

OUTLOOK

Management of Acne Scars in Asian skin

Management of postacne scarring in the Asian population does not differ from that of the Caucasians. (Figure 14.9, 14.10) With the chronicity of hyperpigmented postacne scars among our patients, utilization of topical preparations, from the retinoids to a variety of skin-lightening agents, has been a constant part of the treatment modality offered by our dermatologists. Choices vary and would depend on the effectivity and safety of the agent, proven positive response to the patient, experience of the clinician, and cost of the medication.

Modalities chosen in Western countries are similar to that chosen and performed by the dermatologists in Asia. Treatment preferences, which are dependent on several factors, are mostly logistics or cost oriented and dictated mostly by the availability of the machine, expertise of the clinician, and the affordability/

economics of the procedure. The rapid development of new machines and techniques makes the approach disheartening at times, considering the costs involved while opting for such a new technology. As much as the clinician would want to use each and every new development, these may prove impractical (e.g., a new technology that is not yet proven or not approved generally or risk prone), and more, expensive.

Ablative lasers (CO2 and Er: YAG), considered as the gold standard in laser skin resurfacing, have shown a 25% to 90% efficacy for acne scar treatment.(13) Clinical improvements of 30% to 75% can be achieved for patients with superficial atrophic acne scars. This is associated, however, with a significant degree of adverse effects, especially hyperpigmentation, when used in Asians. Postlaser erythema lasts several weeks to months. Postlaser hyperpigmentation is very common and may last up to 18 months. Postlaser hypopigmentation that may develop can be permanent.(14)

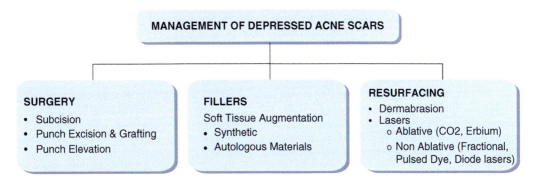

Figure 14.9 Management of Depressed Acne Scars.

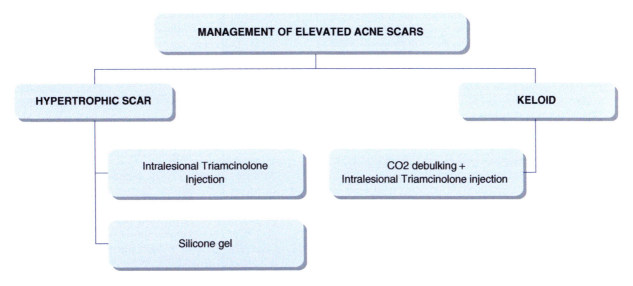

Figure 14.10 Management of Elevated Acne Scars.

Studies were conducted on various approaches on the management of acne scars done among Asians. Experience of Yong-Kwang and Kwok on low fluence-erbium: YAG facial resurfacing was effective and safe in Asian patients (SPT IV-V) with mild-to-moderate severity of atrophic scarring, after only 2 sessions at 1-month interval. Treatment was well tolerated with no postinflammatory hypo- or hyper-pigmentation, neither blistering nor hypertrophic scarring.(15)

Use of nonablative lasers (Nd:YAG 1320 nm or 1064 nm, diode 1450 nm), along with intense pulsed light (IPL) and radiofrequency (RF) devices, is proving to be more applicable in managing the Asian skin and ameliorating the appearance of acne scars without significant downtime but with less efficacy. (16, 17) However, 1450 nonablative diode laser used in Asians with atrophic acne scars provided variable results. In the study done by Chua et al (16); effects were gradual with a 15% to 20% mean improvement achieved after 4 to 6 treatments, but sustained for at least 6 months thereafter. Postlaser hyperpigmentation was significant, hypothesized to be secondary to the sensitivity of darker Asian skin types to cryogen-induced injury and to the high fluence used. Advantages of the procedure, however, were the absence of scarring and hypopigmentation and a minimal postlaser downtime.

The 1320 nm Nd:YAG laser is effective for atrophic acne scar improvement but to further enhance the clinical outcome, a combination approach with another devise such as IPL and a surgical technique such as subcision is necessary.(16)

A total of 27 Asian patients (SPT IV-V) with moderate-to-severe atrophic scarring underwent treatment with 1550 nm erbium-doped fractional photothermolysis (FP) laser for 3 to 5 successive sessions at intervals of 3 to 4 weeks. After only one session, most patients showed visible improvement. Marked improvement in the appearance of acne scars was evident at 3 months post-treatment. The 1550 nm erbium-doped FP is associated with significant patient-reported improvement in the appearance of acne scars with minimal downtime.(17) The results in this study were comparable with those measured by physicians using the long pulsed Er:YAG laser.(19)

For fractional resurfacing, the use of high energy and low density seems to be more appropriate for the treatment of acne scars in Asians.(20, 21) Microdermabrasion and chemical peels are popular among Asians. These are the two top-ranking procedures usally followed by Filipino dermatologists as well. More often than not, the patients are very knowledgeable about these procedures and come to the clinics requesting for such treatment modalities. Though microdermabrasion and chemical peels are being used more often for superficial acne scarring, Chua et al. (18) claimed that these nonlaser treatment modalities generally result in only minimal improvement of superficial atrophic acne scars with poor overall patient satisfaction.

Intralesional injection of glucocorticoids and silicone dressing are regularly used for hypertrophic scars. Ablative skin resurfacing with CO2 laser or Er:YAG and nonablative 585-nm pulsed-dye laser (PDL) are being utilized for less responsive cases. Previously used cryosurgery and radiation are less popular in dealing with this type of acne scar.

SUMMARY

Scarring is an unfortunate complication of acne vulgaris not only among Asians but also among the general population. Understanding of the pathophysiology of acne and its sequela of postacne scarring is essential. Early and aggressive treatment is, therefore, vital to minimize if not prevent its occurrence.

Management of postacne scarring remains a challenge and multiple modalities are often necessary. Individualized approach is crucial to maximize the benefits of various treatment options. With the advent of research and technology, the goal of attaining excellent results in improving acne scars may ultimately be achievable.

REFERENCES

1. Leenutaphong V. Relationship between skin color and cutaneous response to ultraviolet radiation in Thai. Photodermatol Photoimmunol 1995;11:198–203.
2. Youn JI, Oh JK, Kim BK et al. Relation between skin phototype and MED in Korean brown skin. Photodermatol Photoimmunol 1997;13:208–11.
3. Kawasa A. UVB-induced erythema delayed tanning and UVA-induced immediate tanning in Japanese skin. Photodermatol 1986;3:327–33.
4. Verallo-Rowell VM. Understanding the multi-heritage Asian –Filipino Skin Phototype. In: Verallo-Rowell, VM. Skin in the Tropics, Anvil Publishing Philippines, 2001.
5. Goh CL, Akarapanth R. Epidemiology of skin disease among children in a referral skin clinic in Singapore. Pediatr Dermatol 1994;11:125–8.
6. Yeung CK, Teo LH, Xiang LH, Chan HH. A community-based epidemiological study of acne vulgaris in Hong Kong adolescents. Acta Derm Venereol 2002;82:104–7.
7. Sultzberger MB, Zaidems SH. Psychogenic factors in dermatological disorders. Med Clin North Am 1948;32:669.
8. Taylor SC, Cook-Bolden F, Rahman Z et al. Acne vulgaris in skin of color. J Am Acad Dermatol 2002;46:S98–106.
9. Abedeen SK, Gonzalez M, Judodihardjo M, et al. Racial variation in sebum excretion rate. Program and abstracts of the 58th Annual Meeting of the American Academy of Dermatology; March 10-15, 2000; San Francisco, Ca.
10. Zaenglein AL, Graber EM, Thiboutot DM et al. Acne vulgaris and acneiform eruptions. In: Freedberg I, Eisen A, Wolff K, et al. Fitzpatrick's Dermatology in General Medicine 7th ed., Vol 2 McGraw –Hill Co, 2008.
11. Chan HHL. Effective and safe use of lasers, light sources, and radiofrequency devices in the clinical management of Asian patients with selected dermatoses. Lasers Surg Med 2005;37:179–85.

12. Rivera A. Acne scarring: a review and current treatment modalities. J Am Acad Dermatol 2008;59:659–76.

13. Jordan R, Cummins C, Burls A. Laser resurfacing of the skin for the improvement of facial acne scarring: a systematic review of the evidence. Br J Dermatol 2000;142:413–23.

14. Goh CL, Khoo L. Laser skin resurfacing treatment outcome of facial scars and wrinkles in Asians with skin type 3 – 4 with the Unipulse CO2 laser system. Singapore Med J 2002;43:28–32.

15. Yong-Kwang T, Kwok C. Minimally ablative erbium:YAG laser resurfacing of facial atrophic acne scars in Asian skin: a pilot study.Dermatol Surg 2008;34:681–85.

16. Chan HHL, Lam LK, Wong DSY et al. Use of 1320nm Nd: YAG laser for wrinkle reduction and the treatment of atrophic acne scarring in Asians. Lasers Surg Med 2004; 34:98–103.

17. Lee HS, Lee JH, Ahn GY et al. Fractional photothermolysis for the treatment of acne scars: a report of 27 Korean patients. J Dermatol Treatm 2008;19:45–9.

18. Chua SH, Ang P, Khoo LSW et al. Nonablative 1450nm diode laser in the treatment of facial atrophic acne scars in type IV to V Asian skin: A prospective clinical study. Dermatol Surg 2004;30:1287–91.

19. Jeong JT, Kye YC. Resurfacing of pitted facial acne scars with a long pulsed Er:YAG laser. Dermatol Surg 2001;27:107–10.

20. Chan HH, Manstein D, Yu CS et al. The prevalence and risk factors of post inflammatory hyperpigmentation after fractional resurfacing in Asians. Lasers Surg Med 2007;39:381–5.

21. Kono T, Chan HH, Groff WF. Prospective direct comparison study of fractional resurfacing using different fluences and densities for skin rejuvenation in Asians. Lasers Surg Med 2007;39:311–14.

15   Acne scarring and patients of African descent
Ravneet R Kaur, Saba M Ali, and Amy J McMichael

KEY POINTS

- Acne is a common problem among all races and ethnicities. Darker-skinned individuals are at increased risk for postinflammatory hyperpigmentation (PIH) and hypertrophic scarring such as keloids.
- In patients of African descent it is important to consider both aggressive, early prevention of inflammatory acne lesions and treatments that do not induce excessive skin irritation and subsequent postinflammatory hyperpigmentation.
- Types of Scarring: ice pick, rolling, boxcar, and hypertrophic/keloid scarring.
- Medical management of scars: retinoids, topical/injectable steroids, silicone dressing, various other topical or injectable substances.
- Surgical management of scars: punch excision, elliptical excision, punch elevation, skin graft, "subcision," and debulking.
- Procedural management of scars: cryosurgery, electrodesiccation, radiation treatment, chemical peels, microdermabrasion, dermabrasion, tissue augmentation, Laser Therapies: CO_2, Erbium.

INTRODUCTION

Acne is a common disorder affecting up to 45 million people in the United States (1) with a prevalence of 80% in people between 11 and 30 years of age and occurring in 5% of older adults.(2, 3) It is the skin disease most commonly treated by physicians (3) and occurs in people of all ethnicities and races. Currently it is accepted that the pathophysiology, presentation, and treatment of acne are similar in all skin phenotypes. However, acne in pigmented skin is distinguished by the higher incidence of postinflammatory hyperpigmentation and scarring. This chapter will focus on these two major acne sequelae occurring primarily in individuals of African descent.

Acne scarring and postinflammatory hyperpigmentation can have significant psychosocial impact on patients. Scarring can lead to emotional debilitation, embarrassment, poor self-esteem, social isolation, depression, and many other effects.(4) Although these effects cannot be easily quantified in patient terms, healthcare affect, or social expense, scarring is a significant issue that requires attention especially in darker-skinned individuals, as the incidence rates for hypertrophic scarring are higher in this population.(5, 6)

EPIDEMIOLOGY

As the population of the world becomes increasingly diverse, understanding ethnic and racial differences in dermatologic disease is becoming increasingly important. Genetic, environmental, socioeconomic, and cultural factors are likely to contribute to these differences.(7) Currently, there is still a paucity of reliable studies investigating racial and ethnic differences in the epidemiology of dermatologic disease.(6) Most of the data we have is based on practice surveys and individual clinical experience.(7, 8) Neither race nor ethnicity greatly influences acne prevalence. Most surveys show that this skin disorder consistently ranks as the top dermatologic diagnosis in populations of all skin types.(6–8)

Based on a retrospective chart review conducted between August 2004 and July 2005, the six most common diagnoses observed in Black patients were acne, dyschromia, contact dermatitis, and other eczema, alopecia, seborrheic dermatitis, and lesion of unspecified behavior.(7) This study also found that dermatologic visits for acne were the most common in both Black (28.4%) and White (21.0%) patients.(7)

Postinflammatory hyperpigmentation (PIH) is a major acne sequelae in skin of color. In a survey of 2,000 Black patients seen by dermatologists, PIH was the third most common dermatosis seen in 9% of patients (acne 28% and eczema 20%) versus 2% of White patients.(8, 9) A high rate of PIH was also documented in a 2002 survey of African American, Hispanic, and Asian patients. Acne and hyperpigmented macules were found in 65%, 53%, and 47%, of these populations, respectively.(10) It is clear that even though the incidence of acne is fairly equivalent among different skin phototypes, the postinflammatory hyperpigmentation of acne is a much larger concern for patients of color than for White patients.(6, 11)

Hypertrophic and keloidal scarring is not as common as PIH; however, it is more frequent in skin of color and can be more permanent and disfiguring. Keloidal overgrowths of scar tissue are seen between 5 and 16 times more frequently in patients of color.(12) These lesions can be very persistent and are equal in incidence among both sexes. They are less common in the very young or old. Familial and genetic influences with both autosomal dominant and recessive traits are associated with these lesions.(5, 12)

The morbidity of acne is mainly due to the lesions themselves, which may be painful and tender, as well as from residual scarring and postinflammatory hyperpigmentation after the nodules and cysts resolve. Morbidity may be generated by adverse effects of treatments as well. There can be a huge impact on quality of life, especially in terms of psychological morbidity. An estimated $100 million per year is spent on over-the-counter remedies by consumers for acne. When the loss of productivity and unemployment are included the direct cost of acne may exceed $1 billion per year in the United States.(1).

HISTORY

Postinflammatory hyperpigmentation and scarring are the two most disfiguring sequelae of inflammatory acne.(6) The use of topical applications of substances to treat dyspigmentation has existed for centuries. The ancient Egyptians applied animal oils, salt, alabaster, and sour milk to the skin for aesthetic improvement.(13) Dermatologists have continued to advance on these earlier treatments. It was dermatologists who pioneered skin peeling for therapeutic benefit. As early as 1871, Fox, a dermatologist was treating pigmentary changes using Phenol for the treatment of freckles.(14)

Over the years, there have been many attempts to improve acne scarring as well. Ablative techniques such as deep chemical peels, dermabrasion, and more recently, laser-driven skin-resurfacing procedures with CO_2 and/or Er:YAG as well as fractionated lasers have been used.(15) The cosmetic potential of laser therapy was first noticed as a byproduct of early laser treatments of acne.(15, 16) Ablative procedures such as laser treatment have been attempted for scar revision since the 1980s.(17)

POSTINFLAMMATORY HYPERPIGMENTATION

Pathophysiology

Postinflammatory hyperpigmentation represents the skin's response to any type of trauma or cutaneous injury and is often the major sequela of acne. It is visibly more pronounced in darker-skinned individuals. Postinflammatory hyperpigmentation can be either epidermal or dermal. Acne typically results in the epidermal form of hyperpigmentation in which there is an increase in melanin production and/or transfer to keratinocytes.(18) Various inflammatory mediators such as prostaglandins E2 and D2 have been shown to enhance pigment production in animal models and may have a similar role in humans.(18)

The development of postinflammatory hyperpigmentation in the setting of acne may be multifactorial. The lesions of acne itself, including comedones, papules, pustules, and nodules induce hyperpigmentation, but physical manipulation of lesions by the patient or over aggressive, irritating acne treatment regimens can trigger this unwanted skin reaction.

In general, comedonal acne in White skin is characterized as noninflammatory. In biopsies of comedonal acne in Black skin, comedonal lesions exhibit marked inflammation with infiltrates of polymorphonuclear leukocytes.(19) This disparity in histological inflammation between Black skin and White skin helps explain the propensity for darker-skinned individuals to develop postinflammatory hyperpigmentation.

Clinical Features

For many dark-skinned patients, postinflammatory hyperpigmentation (PIH) is more aesthetically unacceptable than the original acne lesions. Subsequently macular hyperpigmentation of the face is often the chief complaint of the acne patient with dark skin when presenting to the dermatologist.

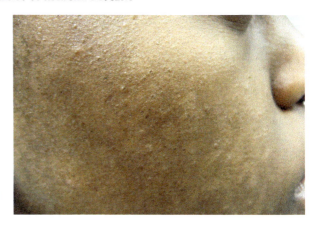

Figure 15.1 Postinflammatory hyperpigmentation from acne.

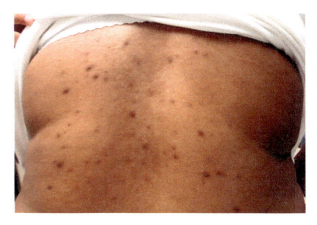

Figure 15.2 Back acne with postinflammatory hyperpigmentation from papular/nodular acne.

PIH presents as asymptomatic tan to dark-brown patches or macules corresponding to the areas of injury (Figure 15.1). The discoloration typically outlasts the acne lesions themselves and can persist for months to years and consequently poses a lingering problem for the patient. In a survey of 239 African Americans with acne, 27.2% tried using over-the-counter 1% to 2% hydroquinone preparations prior to presentation to the dermatologist.(20) Another report states 80% of African patients with acne use skin-lightening agents.(21) Agents commonly employed by patients for the purpose of skin lightening include various over-the-counter acne washes, vinegar, cocoa butter, and hydroquinone; clearly PIH is a major sequela mandating treatment (see Figure 15.2).

Treatment

Essentially, treatment options for acne in white skin and pigmented skin are the same. Topical and systemic retinoids and

Table 15.1 Therapeutic agents for hyperpigmentation.

Mild
    Hydroquinone 2%, 3%, and 4%
    Azelaic Acid 20%
    Kojic Acid 2%-4%
    Tretinoin
    Glycolic Acid

Moderate
    Hydroquinone 4%-10%
    Kojic Acid
    Combination Therapies
        Azelex/Tretinoin
        Hydroquinone/Tretinoin
        Hydroquinone/Glycolic Acid
    Chemical Peels
        Salicylic Acid 20%-30%
        Glycolic Acid 20%-70%
    Trichloracetic Acid 15%-20%

Severe
    Combination Therapies
    Chemical Peels

antibiotics as well as other agents are at the disposal of the dermatologist (Table 15.1). In using these agents, the dermatologist must set expectations for the patient. Advising the parent prior to commencing treatment that it will take 3 months or more to improve postinflammatory hyperpigmentation will help the patient remain compliant with treatment.

In pigmented skin, early and aggressive treatment of acne is of prime importance in preventing complications of postinflammatory hyperpigmentation (PIH). Maximizing initial acne treatment is perhaps the best treatment for PIH. It is equally important to avoid overaggressive, irritating regimens as this can induce PIH. Recognition of the patient's skin type, that is, dry/sensitive skin prone to irritation, normal skin with minimal propensity for irritation, oily skin, or combination skin can aid in choosing an appropriate regimen with the least amount of irritation.(20) In addition, many patients consider their skin "sensitive." It is important to determine what "sensitive" means and if there are true allergies, irritant reactions, or simply dryness in response to treatment.

The retinoids, such as tretinoin, adapalene, and tazarotene, represent a class of topicals that not only treat acne but also hyperpigmentation and, therefore, should be initiated early in treatment and remain as maintenance therapy. It is beneficial to explain to the patient the dual role of retinoids in treatment of acne and hyperpigmentation to foster improved adherence. Retinoids are not only well known for their effect on noninflammatory and inflammatory acne but they can also directly affect postinflammatory hyperpigmentation in dark-skinned individuals.(22–24)

Irritation is a well-documented adverse effect with this class of medications in all skin types. In pigmented skin, minimizing this predictable adverse effect rests on choosing the right vehicle, starting with lower concentrations, considering alternate

day dosing, proper patient education on use, and selecting a tolerable formulation.

Azelaic acid, a dicarboxylic acid obtained from Pityrosporum ovale, is another topical that acts on inflammatory and noninflammatory lesions and hyperpigmentation. It inhibits melanin synthesis by interfering with tyrosinase and has direct cytotoxic effects on melanocytes. It has no effect on normally pigmented skin and is considered to have a low irritancy profile, so may be useful in those with sensitive skin and a history of postinflammatory hyperpigmentation. It can be used in combination with retinoids.

Some individuals, especially those with prominent postinflammatory hyperpigmentation, will also require skin-lightening agents in addition to the traditional acne regimen to combat hyperpigmentation. Hydroquinone, a hydroxylphenol, has been the gold standard for treatment of hyperpigmentation for over 50 years.(25) It reduces the production of melanin by inhibiting tyrosinase, which is responsible for converting DOPA to melanin. Other mechanisms of action, including destruction of melanocytes, degradation of melanosomes, and inhibition of DNA and RNA synthesis, have been attributed to hydroquinone. It is available in over-the-counter concentrations of 1% to 2%, with a prescription strength of 3% to 4% and compounded at 5% to 10%. It is recommended to begin treatment after the acne is under control, or even after 2 to 4 weeks of acne treatment and should be applied after application of topical acne medication. Treatment can be used as spot treatment or diffusely once to twice a day. Results may be noticed within 8 to 12 weeks.(6) Adverse effects include irritant and allergic dermatitis, temporary hypopigmentation of surrounding normal skin giving a halo appearance, and the much-debated exogenous ochronosis with prolonged use. Instruction on how to apply the hydroquinone product over an entire cosmetic unit will help to avoid the localized halo side effect. Various formulations are available; some with additives such as glycolic acid, tretinoin, vitamin C, steroids, sunscreens, and microsponges enhance delivery and efficacy of hydroquinone.(26)

There are numerous other skin-lightening agents available and may be used as alternatives to hydroquinone. A few of these agents will be briefly mentioned here: Mequinol, also known as 4-hydroxyanisole, methoxyphenol, hydroquinone monomethyl ether, and p-hydroxyanisole, is approved in the United States and Europe and is the primary prescription alternative to hydroquinone.(26) The exact mechanism of action is unknown. It does not damage melanocytes, unlike hydroquinone.

Kojic acid, a naturally occurring fungal derivative, is used increasingly in Japan, for treatment of hyperpigmentation. It is available over the counter. It also inhibits tyrosinase by binding to copper, with a reported efficacy similar to over-the-counter hydroquinone.(25)

Arbutin, available over the counter, is a derivative of hydroquinone used in PIH. Obtained from the leaves of the bearberry

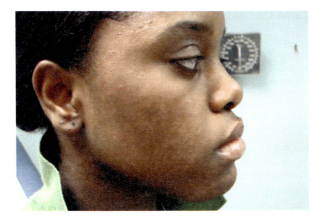

Figure 15.3 Acne with postinflammatory hypopigmentation with pitted scarring.

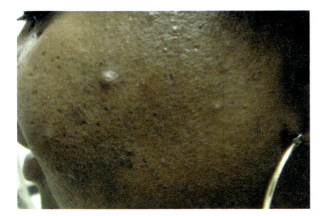

Figure 15.4 Pitted acne scarring in dark skin.

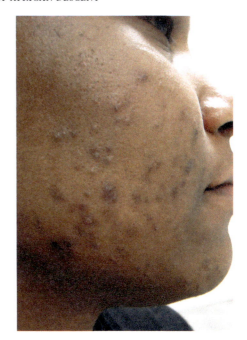

Figure 15.5 Late stage acne scars with fibrous change.

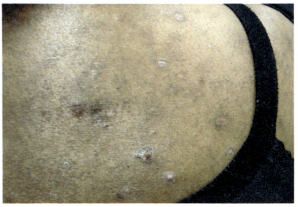

Figure 15.6 Back acne with scarring.

plant, it decreases tyrosinase activity and inhibits melanosome maturation.

Aleosin is a glycoprotein derived from aloe vera that inhibits tyrosinase without cytotoxicity. It has limited ability to penetrate the skin because of its hydrophilic property. It is commonly used with Arbutin.

Licorice extract is considered the safest pigment-lightening agent.(26) Its mechanism of action is similar to kojic acid. The main component is glabridin.

A number of cosmeceutical pigment-lightening agents are available with varying effects and these include N-acetyl glucosamine, soybean trypsin inhibitor, and ascorbic acid. Other options for treating PIH include chemical peels and microdermabrasion. These two modalities will be addressed later in this chapter.

The treatment of hyperpigmentation can be a long, arduous process even with treatment, requiring patience and compliance. Realistic goals must be discussed with the patient.

Daily use of sunscreen and sun protection is an essential component for prevention of PIH and must be stressed to the patient.

ACNE HYPERTROPHIC AND ATROPHIC SCARRING

Clinical Features

Acne scar formation can be broadly divided into two categories: (1) scars as a result of increased tissue formation—hypertrophic and keloid scars, or (2) the more common cause, atrophic scars, which leads to loss or damage of tissue.

ing1ACNE SCARS

Pathophysiology

Unlike atrophic scarring (see Figures 15.3 and 15.4), hypertrophic scarring (see Figures 15.5 and 15.6) and keloids are more common in people of African descent. Keloids are unique to humans and can be described as a disproportionate formation and excess deposition of collagen outside the margins of the original injury.(5) Common locations include the chest, back, shoulders, and ears. Clinically, there may be pain, itching, burning, or limited range of motion. Histology shows a normal-appearing dermis with relaxed, randomly aligned collagen. Both hypertrophic scars and keloids demonstrate thicker, more abundant collagen that is stretched and aligned in the same plane as the epidermis. Islands of dermal collagen fibers, small vasculature, and fibroblasts can be seen throughout hypertrophic scars.(27) Suggested pathophysiology includes a variety of different factors such as altered microvascular regeneration, transforming growth factor-beta-I, interleukin-I-alpha, platelet-derived growth factor, matrix metalloproteinases, fibroblasts themselves, histamine, carboxypeptidase A, prostaglandin D2, and tryptase.(28) Keloids are different in that they are more acellular than hypertrophic scars and have reticular dermal acellular node-like structures.(5) In vitro studies show that keloid fibroblasts continue to produce high levels of collagen, fibronectin, elastin, and proteoglycan, and show aberrant responses, compared with normal fibroblasts, to metabolic modulators such as glucocorticoids, hydrocortisone, and growth factors.(28)

Treatment of Acne Scars

Treating acne scars can be one of the most difficult cosmetic surgery procedures that exists.(29) The difficulty in achieving total correction of damage caused by severe inflammatory acne is that the epidermis, dermis, and underlying fat are often involved. The goal of treatment should be to obtain as much improvement as possible rather than perfection.(30) Medical, surgical, and procedural options will be discussed for the management of scarring.

MEDICAL MANAGEMENT OF SCARRING

Inflammatory cysts and nodules can be extremely tender and painful. In ethnic skin, they can evolve into keloids and other hypertrophic scar.(31) Medical management focuses on the treatment of pigmentary changes, hypertrophic scars, and keloids. Other types of scarring require other forms of intervention. Retinoids, topical/injectable steroids, and silicone dressings are the most commonly used and accepted in the medical management of acne scarring (Table 15.2).

There are a myriad of other possible topical and injectable substances that have been examined in the treatment of acne scars but will not be discussed in depth. These include antioxidants, zinc, colchicine, hyaluronidase, cyclosporine, honey, onion extract, 5-fluorouracil, bleomycin, retinoids, verapamil, pepsin, hydrochloric acid, formalin, and many others.(5)

There are a few reports of treatment of keloids, hypertrophic scars, and very superficial scars with retinoids.(32) The benefit

Table 15.2 Medical management.

Retinoids
Topical/injectable steroids
Silicone dressing
Various other topical or injectable substances

of retinoid treatment is attributed to an increase in elasticity with dermal collagen deposition and alignment.(33)

Steroids are another one of the more popular choices for medical therapy for hypertrophic scars and keloids. They have immunomodulatory and antiinflammatory properties and work by reducing the expression of cytokines, cellular adhesion molecules, and other enzymes related to the inflammatory process.(34) The exact mechanism is unknown but the antiinflammatory properties, along with a reduction of collagen, glycosaminoglycans, and fibroblasts, are thought to play a role. Overall retardation of growth of the lesion can also be involved. Clinical responses can be varied as steroids can be used topically with and without occlusion. Possible side effects of topical steroids are well known and include telangiectasias, bruising, atrophy, pain, or pigmentary change.

Intralesional steroid injections are another route; some recommend injections as first-line treatment for hypertrophic scars and keloids because surgery is often debatable for these lesions. A multiple-modality treatment is recommended due to the high recurrence with surgery alone. Surgery is often performed for debulking; aggressive scars have a regrowth rate of 50% to 100%.(5) To prevent acne scarring, cystic nodules can be directly injected with triamcinolone acetonide (2.5–5.0 mg/cc via 1-cc syringe and 30-G needle). Resolution usually occurs within 2 to 5 days. To flatten keloids, a higher concentration of the corticosteroid (e.g., 10 to 20 mg/cc) should be used. Repeat injections can be given every 2 to 4 weeks.(6) With intralesional injections, often multiple injections spaced one or several months apart are required to determine the final result and prevent excess atrophy.(5) Intralesional steroids can also be used to create atrophy in an area where there has been an overcorrection with permanent filler for augmentation. Other side effects of injected steroids include intolerance, necrosis, allergy, bruising, hyperpigmentation or hypopigmentation, injection pain, and telangiectasias. Of these side effects hypopigmentation can be a major concern for patients of color. Minimizing the amount of steroid injected, selecting a few lesions for trial, and spacing injections by at least 4 weeks can help prevent hypopigmentation. Choosing lesions that are located in inconspicuous areas for the first treatment may also give an idea of how the skin will respond to a given concentration of injected steroid.

Silicone dressings are another treatment option for hypertrophic scars and to a lesser extent for keloids. These are completely safe to use in darker skin types, although there are variable results with this treatment modality. The results are likely attributable to occlusion or hydration. Pressure, temperature, increased oxygen tension, electrostatic properties, and immunologic effects have

Table 15.3 Surgical management.

Punch Excision
Elliptical Excision
Punch Elevation
Skin graft
Subcision
Debulking

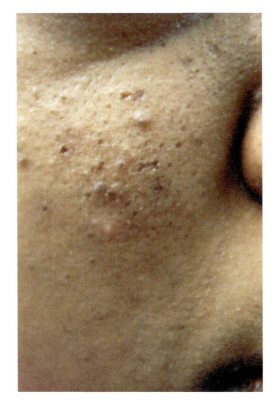

Figure 15.7 Boxcar scars and rolling scars from facial acne.

all been other rationales for the use of silicone dressings. There are conflicting reports as to its efficacy.(5) In one randomized control trial an improvement in pruritus, pain, and pliability was reported, but no improvement in pigmentation, average elevation, or minimum elevation of scars was found.(35) Another review of effects, efficacy, and safety determined that side effects rarely occur but can include pruritus, contact dermatitis, maceration, skin breakdown, xerosis, and odor.(5)

In terms of ease of use, silicone dressings do not suit facial scars well since they would be visible to others if worn in public. Thus, these dressings may best serve large areas on the chest or back that can easily be camouflaged with clothing. Another worry with these dressings is that most studies support their use in early forming scars as opposed to late scars.(5)

SURGICAL MANAGEMENT OF SCARRING

Surgical management of acne scarring is one of the mainstays of treatment in lighter skin types. However, caution must be used when applying surgical approaches to darker skin types due to the propensity of developing further scarring. A single typical lesion can be treated to observe the outcome before proceeding with a full face of scars. Also, less visible scars along the hair line or ears can be treated first to make sure the resultant scar from treatment is both acceptable and an improvement over the original scar. If a surgical treatment is performed, close follow-up with bleaching agents and/or intralesional steroid is prudent.

Ice-pick, boxcar, and rolling scars are frequently addressed by surgery (Table 15.3 and Figure 15.7). Each type of scar has an optimal method by which it can be improved. Ice-pick scars are usually smaller in diameter (<2 mm) and deep with possible tracts to the dermis or subcutaneous tissue. These are commonly seen on the cheeks. Treatment is frequently performed by punch excision.(2) Nonabsorbable suture is preferred secondary to the predisposition to scar.(36) Elliptical excision to the subcutaneous level is the other preferred technique for ice-pick scars.

Skin grafts are rarely required. Punch elevation is another method of treating acne scars. Punch elevation combines the techniques of punch excision and grafting without the risk of skin color or texture mismatch.(2) This is often the treatment for depressed boxcar scars. It is essential that the biopsy tool exactly matches the inner diameter of the lesion.(5, 2) The base should sit slightly higher than the surrounding skin. Retraction of the grafted tissue occurs during the healing phase, resulting in a leveled surface. The "floating" punched specimen is affixed

to the surrounding tissue. After the punch is done and the base elevated, it is sutured flush with the normal-appearing skin and allowed to heal in place. This is routinely performed with either sutures or Steri-Strips.(37)

Lastly, the surgical choice for rolling or depressed scars is "subcision." This technique of subcutaneous incision or "subcision" is generally considered safe to use in black skin. The goal is to free the tethering fibrous bands that cause rolling scars. A tri-bevel needle is probed under the lesion through the needle's puncture so it is not a true incision. The movement of triangular tip of the needle results in the releasing of papillary skin from the binding connections of the deeper tissues. This creates a controlled trauma that leads to wound healing and associated additional connective tissue formation in the treated location. Uncommonly, there is the potential for bruising, hypertrophy, cysts from pilosebaceous unit disruption, infection, additional scar, or worsening of the scar.(5) The use of filler substances in conjunction with subcision can also be performed.(2)

Most often, keloid and hypertrophic scars are treated with medical management. If an attempt is made to excise a keloid, close follow-up and treatment with intralesional corticosteroids are necessary. The goal is more to reduce overall size or debulk rather than completely excise the keloidal or hypertrophic scar.

Table 15.4 Procedural management.

Cryosurgery
Electrodessication
Radiation treatment
Chemical peels
Microdermabrasion
Dermabrasion

Secondary, refining procedures can also been used when desired or needed. Such procedures include laser skin resurfacing after punch excision, as well as all of the medical and procedural options after any surgical management. There are few studies looking at the safety and efficacy of laser skin resurfacing in darker skin types. Thus, in general practice it is not considered first-line treatment because of the risks of hypopigmentation and PIH postprocedure.

PROCEDURAL MANAGEMENT OF SCARRING

Several procedural options will be covered within this section (Table 15.4). Cryosurgery for hypertrophic scars and electrodessication for boxcar scars are two simple procedural treatment options (30) that are not often used in darker-skinned patients, as there is an increased risk of permanent atrophy, hypopigmentation, or creation of a new scar.(5)

Radiation can be used for hypertrophic and keloidal scars. It causes destruction of fibroblast vasculature, a decrease in fibroblast activity, and induces local cellular apoptosis.(38) This modality is used more as an adjunct to prevent a recurrence as opposed to a stand-alone treatment.(5) In Japan, 38 keloids (ear, neck, and upper lip) were treated with surgical excision followed by electron-beam radiation within a few days. There was a significant improvement of pigmentation, pliability, height, vascularity, and hardness. Recurrence rate was 21.2% overall with no recurrences observed in the craniofacial area. The results of this trial are applicable for patients who have a Fitzpatrick skin type of III or greater.(39) Risks from radiation include hyperpigmentation or hypopigmentation, prolonged erythema, telangiectasias, atrophy, and questionable increase in malignancies.(5) Chemical peels can also be used to address the residual scarring from acne lesions. These peels can vary in depth of penetration from superficial to deep. Unless the very deep peels are used, these are generally considered useful for milder acne scarring but certainly not ice-pick or keloid scars. Usually multiple treatments are necessary for efficacy. These treatment modalities are also useful for the treatment of PIH seen in darker skinned patients. Postprocedure, patients can expect a mild desquamation with normal skin regeneration.

A variety of superficial chemical peels are available, including beta hydroxyl acid (salicylic) 20% to 30%; alpha hydroxyl acid (glycolic, lactic, or citric) 20% to 70%; Jessner's peel, trichloroacetic acid 15% to 30%; a combination of glycolic acid and trichloroacetic acid, and resorcinol.(5, 40–43) Considerations when choosing a peel include the concentration, duration, skin type, prior medical or surgical intervention, location, sun exposure pre- and postprocedure, concomitant medications, and other factors.

In dark-complexioned patients, a transient PIH is not uncommon, especially following a stronger peeling course. When the salicylic acid peel is carefully titrated at 20% to 30%, it has been shown to be safe and effective in ethnic skin.(44) Beta hydroxy acids inhibit the arachidonic pathway and, therefore, decrease inflammation and may be better for easily irritated skin and are well known to be safer in darker skin types.(43)

Chemical peels should be started at a lower concentration and titrated upward as tolerated in darker-skinned patients to limit irritant contact dermatitis and PIH. The peel can be performed at 2- to 4-week intervals. Patients should be advised to discontinue retinoid therapy 5 to 7 days prior to each peel.(16) The treatment-induced PIH can be minimized with a hydroquinone pre- and posttreatment within 7 to 10 days of the peel. The other types of chemical peels have increased risks in darker-skinned patients and are used less often.

An important study introducing the CROSS (chemical reconstruction of skin scars) method for dark-complexioned patients (Fitzpatrick skin types IV-V), used TCA at high concentrations applied directly to scars. After 3 to 6 treatments, 90% of patients showed good (50%–70%) improvement by blinded physician assessment. Within the 65% TCA group, 82% were satisfied with results compared with 94% satisfaction in the 100% TCA group. They found the technique to be safe, with the 100% TCA treatments of atrophic scars more effective than the 65% TCA treatments.(41)

Two other management options utilize direct mechanical means of skin removal. Microdermabrasion provides more of a texture benefit than permanent surface change and may address the epidermal component of acne-related PIH as well as problems related to skin texture and enlarged pores.(6, 45) Studies with microdermabrasion are few in patients with ethnic skin.(16, 46) Thus, at present, the procedure should be considered mainly for patients who are sensitive to the chemicals used in peels.(16) Several treatment sessions are typically required and retinoids should be discontinued 3 to 5 days before the procedure. Posttreatment PIH is a concern and hydroquinone can be continued between treatments. The most improvement is achieved in PIH, although superficial acne scars may benefit from deeper, more aggressive settings.(45) Side effects can typically include temporary stripping of the treatment area; bruising, burning, or stinging sensation; photosensitivity; and occasional pain. Patients using isotretinoin should wait up to 6 months after the last ingestion to minimize side effects.(5) Dermabrasion is infrequently performed in darker phototypes due to the very high risk of pigmentary alteration and scarring.(16)

TISSUE AUGMENTATION

For patients with few scars, augmentation is another alternative for the management of acne scarring. The past decade has seen the advent of a multitude of injectable, fillers including human collagen, polylactic acid, and hyaluronic acid among the short-term agents and many agents of a longer-term nature with the reintroduction of silicone and variations of polyacrylamides for longer correction. Agents may be xenografts, autografts, homografts, or synthetics.(47) For those with few scars, simple dermal augmentation with bovine or human collagen (Zyderm and Cosmoderm, Inamed Aesthetics, Santa Barbara, CA) or hyaluronic acid (Restylane, Medicis, Scottsdale, AZ; Juvederm and Hylaform; Inamed Aesthetics) would be most appropriate. In patients with limited acne scarring overcorrection should be avoided.

There are few to no studies that specifically examine the use of filler agents in skin of color. The safety and use of Restylane, a hyaluronic acid, have been studied in patients with Fitzpatrick skin types IV to VI in isolated cases. There were no transient or permanent adverse outcomes among the type IV to VI subjects in those cases. If proper injection techniques are used, patients with Fitzpatrick skin types IV to VI can benefit from this hyaluronic acid product.(48)

LIGHT, LASER AND ENERGY THERAPY IN ACNE SCAR ABLATION

When using light and lasers in the treatment of acne scarring, there is a higher risk of side effects in darker-skinned patients because of the nonspecific energy absorption by the relatively large quantities of melanin in the basal layer of the epidermis. These side effects include permanent dyspigmentation, textural changes, focal atrophy, and scarring. Epidermal melanin can also compete for absorption of energy and decrease the total amount of energy reaching deeper dermal lesions. It is imperative to consider power level as well as the wavelength of the laser when treating darker skin. Power setting should be conservative (the minimal threshold fluences necessary to produce the desired tissue effect in a given individual). Test spots should be performed whenever possible. In treating darker skin, it is always best to err on the side of caution rather than risk excessive thermal injury. All of this makes it more difficult to achieve the desired clinical result.(49, 50) The absorption coefficient of melanin decreases exponentially as wavelengths increase.(51) Therefore, to produce a safer laser system, it needs to generate wavelengths that are less efficiently absorbed by endogenous melanin but can still achieve the desired results.(52)

Cutaneous laser resurfacing can be an effective approach for improving the appearance of atrophic scarring in patients with darker skin phototypes (Table 15.5). Several reports document the long-term safety of the high-energy, pulsed, and scanned carbon dioxide (CO2), and short- and long-pulsed erbium:yttrium–aluminum garnet (Er:YAG) lasers for the treatment of more darkly pigmented patients. Skin resurfacing with the CO_2 laser remains the gold-standard technology for production of the most dramatic clinical and histologic improvement in scarred facial skin. Use of the CO_2 laser for skin resurfacing yields an additional benefit of collagen tightening through heating of dermal collagen. To minimize the risk of adverse events, it is best to avoid overlapping or stacking of

Table 15.5 Laser, light, and energy.

Ablative lasers	Nonablative lasers	Light and energy
Carbon-dioxide	532-nm KTP	Intense pulsed light
Er:YAG	510/585-nm Pulsed dye	Radiofrequency
Fractionated (also nonablative)	1064/1320-nm Nd:YAG	Plasma
	1450-nm Diode	
	1540 Er:glass	

Er, Erbium; *KTP*, potassium-titanylphosphate; *Nd*, neodymium; *YAG*, yttrium-aluminum-garnet.

laser scans or pulses. If patients have scarring on their neck or chest, it is best to avoid resurfacing in these areas due to the scarcity of pilosebaceous units in these regions with resultant slow reepithelialization and potential for scarring.(55)

The wavelength of the CO_2 laser is 10,600 nm and the target chromophore is extracellular and intracellular water. There have been a few studies that specifically look at the efficacy and rate of adverse events from ablative CO_2 laser in darker skin types. Often studies will include patients with Fitzpatrick skin type up to V but do not specify the number of patients of each respective phototype that makes it difficult to ascertain the true efficacy and safety of these procedures. Hyperpigmentation is observed in all skin phototypes following CO_2 laser irradiation, however, at a higher incidence in darker skin tones.(56)

The Er:YAG laser attempts to duplicate the results of the CO_2 laser while minimizing the side effects. The wavelength emitted is designed to be absorbed more efficiently and superficially, and the short pulses limit the amount on thermal necrosis. Thus, the Er:YAG is able to provide shorter recovery times, reduced posttreatment erythema, and a decreased risk of dyspigmentation.(57, 58) Similar to the CO2 laser, this laser may benefit hypertrophic scars, rarely keloids, and shallower boxcar scars. The most common side effect post–laser skin resurfacing is transient hyperpigmentation and it affects approximately one-third of all patients. It is important to note that the incidence rises to 68% to 100% among patients with the darkest skin phototypes.(59)

Another study out of Korea was done in exclusively darker-skinned patients (Fitzpatrick skin phototypes III-V) to evaluate the clinical and histologic effects of long-pulsed Er:YAG laser resurfacing for pitted facial acne scars. In this study, 35 patients with pitted facial acne scars were treated with a long-pulsed Er:YAG. The results of long-pulsed Er:YAG laser resurfacing for pitted facial acne scars were excellent in 10 patients (36%), good in 16 patients (57%), and fair in 2 patients (7%). Erythema occurred in all patients after laser treatment and lasted longer than 3 months in 15 patients (54%). Postinflammatory hyperpigmentation occurred in 8 patients (29%). But the pigmentation faded or disappeared within 3 months. No scarring, bacterial infection, or contact dermatitis was observed. This study showed that resurfacing with a long-pulsed Er:YAG laser is a safe and very effective treatment modality for pitted facial acne scars in skin phototypes III-V.(60)

Of particular importance is strict avoidance of excessive sun exposure and the use of a full-spectrum sunblock consistently before and after laser treatment.(61) Some presurgical topical treatments may enhance the eventual postoperative results by decreasing the risk of PIH. There are conflicting opinions regarding pretreatment with hydroquinone, tretinoin, or glycolic acid to decrease the incidence of hyperpigmentation after ablative laser resurfacing in any skin phototype.(62) However, topical tretinoin, hydroquinone, and mild topical steroids are thought to be important postlaser procedure, especially in patients with darker skin.(60)

Retinoic acid topically appears to speed reepithelialization rates, and it can reduce rates of melanin production after the initial stage of healing is completed and the skin can tolerate the retinoic acid.(63) Critical in darker-skinned patients, even if retinoic acid does not decrease the actual incidence of posttreatment PIH, it may reduce its severity and duration.

Another approach is the newer nonablative laser technology that may provide both greater efficacy and safety in patients with darker skin. They have a lower risk of pigmentary alterations when compared to ablative technologies adding to their appeal for use in darker skin types. Nonablative technologies can be laser, light-based, or radiofrequency energies. These modalities are less aggressive, and thus better for the treatment of atrophic, rolling, or possibly hypertrophic scars. A multitude of systems with "subsurfacing" capabilities has been studied, including IPL and pulsed dye, Nd:YAG, diode, and Er:glass lasers.(59) Typically, patients will receive several treatments monthly. These treatments create a controlled thermal injury in the dermis leading to inflammation, cytokine upregulation, and fibroblast proliferation for improvement of scars.

Fractional photothermolysis, a new concept was first introduced and discussed in 2004.(64) It is one of the latest technologies introduced for laser skin resurfacing and treatment of atrophic scars without a significant risk of side effects.(64) It creates minute columns of thermal injury in the dermis called microscopic treatment zones (MTZ) that contain areas of localized epidermal necrosis and collagen denaturation. Rapid healing occurs from the viable epidermal and dermal cells residing in the intact tissue surrounding each MTZ. Because there is selective sparing of skin rather than total ablation, there tend to be less problems overall when compared to the CO_2 laser.(65)

A study of 53 patients (Fitzpatrick I-V) using a 1,550-nm erbium-doped fractional laser on facial skin with mild-to-moderate atrophic acne were treated with several sessions. Blinded assessments of photographs revealed 91% to have 25% to 50% improvement after a single treatment, whereas 87% of patients undergoing 3 treatments had 51% to 75% improvement. Age, sex, and skin type (I-V) did not alter the outcome with maintained results at 6-month follow-up.(66)

The 585-nm pulse-dye laser (PDL) is a nonablative laser to use for hypertrophic scars or keloids. This laser targets erythema and vascularity and is thus better at improving the hyperemia and scar elevation in hypertrophic scars. Because Fitzpatrick

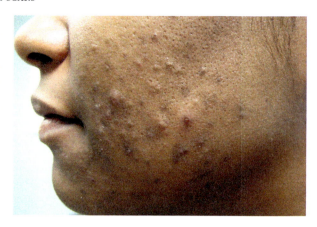

Figure 15.8 Papular and nodular acne with postinflammatory hyperpigmentation.

skin types I or II patients have less competition with melanin they obtain the best results and least side effects. However, in one study patients up to a skin type of IV were found to have significant improvement of their scarring, using this treatment modality. Ten patients (mean age 34.8 years) with Fitzpatrick skin types I-IV with shallow to moderately deep, saucerized facial acne scars had a single laser treatment with a 585-nm PDL to both cheeks. By day 120, all 10 patients reported visible cosmetic improvement while surface profilometry using silicone imprints showed that, on average, the depth of the acne scars was reduced by 47.8%. No adverse effects of this treatment were reported.(67) Another study using the PDL showed a significant increase in the dermal collagen production rate after treatment. The results are postulated to be related to increased fibroblast activity leading to deposition of new collagen in the dermal region of the skin.(68)

The 1,064-nm neodymium:YAG (Nd:YAG) laser. This laser demonstrates greater effect on vasculature than on pigment effect leading to hemostasis and resultant infarctions within vessels. A recent study to evaluate the effectiveness for atrophic scars was done in 12 subjects (age 18–36 years, average age 27.6 years; Fitzpatrick II-V) with mild-to-moderate atrophic acne scars. Patients were treated with the 1,064-nm Nd:YAG laser every 4 to 6 weeks over 8 months, covering a total of 5 sessions. Mild-to-moderate clinical improvement was observed in most patients. One patient developed pitted scars associated with blistering, which occurred 1 to 3 days after the treatment. Because this patient had dark skin, postlaser hyperpigmentation was noted; however, it completely disappeared within 4 months. However, photographic assessment of scars found visible cosmetic improvement in the other 11 patients. All patients were satisfied. There were statistically significant collagen increases in the dermis following the treatment. Side effects were limited to mild, transient erythema and increased skin sensitivity after the procedure. The 1,064-nm Nd:YAG laser may possibly be a safe

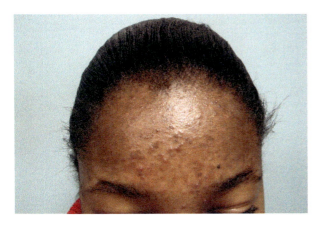

Figure 15.9 Pomade acne on forehead.

and effective nonablative method for improving atrophic scars, even in darker skin but should still be used with caution.(69)

Intense pulsed light (IPL) is not a true laser, but instead these machines emit a wide range of wavelengths from their source that can be precisely narrowed using wavelength filters. Plasma is one of the newest forms of treatment in which ultrahigh radiofrequency energy is passed through inert nitrogen gas.(5) There are currently no studies looking at the use of plasma in darker-skinned individuals. However, because this is a treatment modality using energy rather than a chromophore, there is a potential to use this in darker-skinned individuals in the future. All of these options, in combination, allow for tailoring therapy to a defined goal.

UNIQUE ACNE CONSIDERATIONS IN PIGMENTED SKIN
Nodulocystic acne appears to be less common in people of African descent than in Caucasians and Hispanics. This has been reported in various surveys.(1, 10, 70) Studies have also found that isotretinoin is prescribed less often for African Americans than for Caucasians.(71) There were 35 million visits to physicians for the treatment of acne between 1990 and 1997, and isotretinoin was prescribed at 5.8 million (17%) of these visits. Per capita visit rates for acne among Whites were 2.3 times that of Blacks, and Whites were 1.8 times more likely to receive isotretinoin at acne visits.(72)

Nodulocystic acne has implications for the patient as it is more likely to lead to scarring (see Figure 15.8). A systemic retinoid such as isotretinoin is the treatment of choice for nodulocystic acne in patients with ethnic skin.(6) Still, studies have shown that there is a relatively low usage of isotretinoin among patients of color.(71) Early treatment with isotretinoin in patients of color with moderate or mild acne may be justified in some cases as a way to subvert development of PIH and keloidal scarring.(73) Skin dryness, a common side effect of isotretinoin, is of particular importance to patients of color as it can result in PIH. Emollients and topical corticosteroids can be used to minimize this side effect.(6)

Another unique consideration in African American skin is pomade acne (see Figure 15.9). Pomade acne is related to the use of a thick, oily dressing called pomade or hair grease that can be quite comedogenic.(6) In a survey, almost half of the dark-skinned patients with acne said they used pomades.(10) Pomade is generally used for hair sculpting. Pomade acne occurs in a characteristic distribution on the forehead, and anterior hairline where the hair product comes into contact with the skin. It usually consists of comedones, with perhaps a few papules and pustules and may also cause some inflammation secondary to irritation from chemicals. Often this leads to PIH to the affected areas. Suggestions to decrease the risk of PIH secondary to pomade acne are to (a) apply the pomade 1 inch behind the hairline if using it for scalp dryness; (b) if using the pomade to make the hair more manageable or to create a certain hairstyle, try applying the pomade to the ends only; and lastly (3) simply stop using pomade. Acne should gradually clear if there is no further contact of pomade with the skin. If it persists, the acne should be treated the same as any other acne.(6, 74)

SUMMARY
In treating acne scarring in patients of African descent, prevention of the acne is key. While the deeper pigmentation plays a large role in the PIH observed in this population, all the factors that contribute to scarring in patients of African descent are not known, but are likely further reaching than simple pigmentation. These patients are at increased risk for postinflammatory hyperpigmentation, hypertrophic scarring, and keloids. Treatment of postinflammatory hyperpigmentation and true scars resulting from acne must reflect several considerations by the physician: cost, severity of lesions, physician goals, patient expectations, side-effect profiles, and psychological or emotional effect to the patient. Side-effect profiles must be carefully weighed against benefits, particularly in darker-skinned individuals who may be more prone to adverse reactions to common treatments for acne scarring. Close follow-up, an emphasis on compliance, and counseling regarding the use of noncomedogenic and nonirritating skin and hair care products will aid in yielding better outcomes.(6, 74) Most important, the physician and the patient must agree on realistic treatment goals. As acne scarring is one of the most difficult conditions to treat, especially in darker-skinned individuals, often the goal is improvement, not perfection of acne scarring.

REFERENCES
1. Centers for Disease Control and Prevention. National Center for Health Statistics. National ambulatory medical care survey. http://www.cdc.gov/nchs/about/major/ahcd/namcsdes.htm
2. Jacob CI, Dover JS, Kaminer MS. Acne scarring: a classification system and review of treatment options. J Am Acad Derma 2001; 45: 109–17.
3. Pochi PE. The pathogenesis and treatment of acne. Annu Rev Med 1990; 41: 187–98.

4. Koo J. The psychosocial impact of acne: patients' perceptions. J Am Acad Dermatol 1995; 32(Suppl): S26–30.

5. Rivera A. Acne scarring: a review and current treatment modalities. J Am Acad Dermatol 2008; 59(4): 659–76.

6. Callender, VD. Considerations for treating acne in ethnic skin. Cutis 2005; 76(2 Suppl): 19–23.

7. Alexis AF, Sergay AB. Taylor SC. Common dermatologic disorders in skin of color: a comparative practice survey. Cutis 2007; 80(5): 387–94.

8. Taylor SC. Epidemiology of skin disease in ethnic populations. Dermatol Clin 2003; 21: 601–7.

9. Halder RM, Grimes PE, McLaurin CI, Kress MA, Kenney JA. Incidence of common dermatoses in a predominantly black dermatologic practice. Cutis 1983; 32: 388–90.

10. Taylor SC, Cook-Bolden F, Rahman Z, Strachan D. Acne vulgaris in skin of color. J Am Acad Dermatol 2002; 46(Suppl): S98–S106.

11. McMichael AJ. Diagnosis and treatment of acne vulgaris. Monthly Prescribing Reference. 2004 Edition.

12. Shaffer JJ, Taylor SC, Cook-Bolden F. Keloidal scars: a review with a critical look at therapeutic options. J Am Acad Dermatol 2002: 46(Suppl): S63–S97.

13. Brody HJ, Monheit GD, Resnik SS, Alt TH. A history of chemical peeling. Dermatologic Surgery 2001; 26(5): 405–9.

14. Brody HJ. Variations and comparisons in medium-depth chemical peeling. J Dermatol Surg Oncol 1989; 15: 953–63.

15. Greeley A. Cosmetic laser surgery. FDA Consumer. [WWW document.] URL http://www.fda.gov/fdac/features/2000/300_laser.html (Accessed November 2008).

16. Callender VD. Cosmetic surgery in skin of color. Cosm Derm 2003: 53–6.

17. Sawcer D, Lee HR, Lowe NJ. Lasers and adjunctive treatments for facial scars: a review. J Cutan Laser Ther 1999; 1(2): 77–85.

18. Chang MW. Disorders of hyperpigmentation. In: Bolognia JL, Jorizzo JL, Rapini RP (eds). Dermatology. New York: Mosby, 2008: 947.

19. Halder RM, Holmes YC, Bridgeman-Shah S, Kligman AM. A clinicopathological study of acne vulgaris in black females. J Invest Dermatol 1996; 106: 888.

20. Taylor SC. Skin of color: biology, structure, function, and implications for dermatologic disease. J Am Acad Dermatol 2002; 46(Suppl): S41–S62.

21. Poli F. Acne on pigmented skin. Int J of Dermatol 2007; 46(Suppl 1): 39–41.

22. Jacyk WK, Mpofu P. Adapalene gel 0.1% for topical treatment of acne vulgaris in African patients. Cutis 2001; 68(Suppl 4): 48–54.

23. Bulengo-Ransby SM, Griffiths CE, Kimbrough-Green CK et al. Topical tretinoin (retinoic acid) therapy for hyperpigmented lesions caused by inflammation of the skin in black patients. N Engl J Med 1993; 328: 1438–43.

24. Grimes P, Callender VD. Tazarotene cream for postinflammatory hyperpigmentation and acne vulgaris in darker skin: a double-blind, randomized, vehicle–controlled study. Cutis 2006; 77(1): 45–50.

25. Halder RM, Richards GM. Topical agents used in the management of hyperpigmentation. Skin Therapy Lett 2004; 9(6): 1–3.

26. Draelos ZD. Skin lightening preparations and the hydroquinone controversy. Dermatol Ther 2007; 20(5): 308–13.

27. Tuan TL, Nichter LS. The molecular basis of keloid and hypertrophic scar formation. Mol Med Today 1998; 4: 19–24.

28. Bouzari N, Davis SC, Nouri K. Laser treatment of keloids and hypertrophic scars. Int J Dermatol 2007; **46:** 80–8.

29. Fulton JE. Dermabrasion, chemabrasion and laser abrasion. Dermatol Surg 1996; **22:** 619–28.

30. Kadunc BV, Trindale de Albeida AR. Surgical treatment of facial acne scars based on the morphologic classification: a Brazilian experience. Dermatol Surg 2003; 29: 1200–9.

31. Halder RM. The role of retinoids in management of cutaneous conditions in blacks. J Am Acad Dermatol 1998; 39: S98–103.

32. Harris DW, Buckley CC, Ostler LS, Rustin MHA. Topical retinoic acid in the treatment of fine acne scarring. Br J Dermatol 1991; 125(1): 81.

33. Berardesca E, Gabba P, Farinelli N, Borroni G, Rabbiosi G. In vivo tretinoin-induced changes in skin mechanical properties. Br J Dermatol 1990; 122: 525–9.

34. Jalali M, Bayat A. Current use of steroids in management of abnormal raised skin scars. Surgeon 2007; 5: 175–80.

35. Phillips TJ, Gerstein AD, Lordan V. A randomized controlled trial of hydrocolloid dressing in the treatment of hypertrophic scars and keloids. Dermatol Surg 1996; 22: 775–8.

36. Jemec JB, Jemec B. Acne: treatment of scars. Clin Dermatol 2004; 22: 434–8.

37. Whang KK, Lee M. The principle of a three-staged operation in the surgery of acne scars. J Am Acad Dermatol 1999; 40: 95–7.

38. Doornbos JF, Stoffel TJ, Hass AC et al. The role of kilovoltage irradiation in the treatment of keloids. Int J Radiat Oncol Biol Phys 1990; 18: 833–9.

39. Akita S, Akino K, Yakabe A et al. Combined surgical excision and radiation therapy for keloid treatment. J Craniofac Surg 2007; 18: 1164–9.

40. Al-Waiz MM, Al-Sharqi AI. Medium-depth chemical peels in the treatment of acne scars in dark-skinned individuals. Dermatol Surg 2002; 28: 383–7.

41. Lee JB, Chung WG, Kwahck H, Lee KH. Focal treatment of acne scars with trichloroacetic acid: chemical reconstruction of skin scars method. Dermatol Surg 2002; 28: 1017–21.

42. Wang CM, Huang CL, Hu CT, Chan HL. The effect of glycolic acid on the treatment of acne in Asian skin. Dermatol Surg 1997; 23: 23–9.

43. Burns RL, Prevost-Blank PL, Lawry MA et al. Glycolic acid peels for postinflammatory hyperpigmentation in black patients. A comparative study. Dermatol Surg 1997; 23: 171–4.
44. Grimes PE. The safety and efficacy of salicylic acid chemical peels in darker racial-ethnic groups. Dermatol Surg 1999; 25: 18–22.
45. Savardekar P. Microdermabrasion. Indian J Dermatol Venereol Leprol 2007; 73: 277–9.
46. Rajan P, Grimes PE. Skin barrier changes induced by aluminum oxide and sodium chloride microdermabrasion. Dermatol Surg 2002; 28: 390–3.
47. Klein AW. Skin filling: collagen and other injectables of the skin. Dermatol Clin 2001; 19: 491–508.
48. Odunze M, Cohn A, Few JW. Restylane in people of color. Plast Reconstr Surg 2007; 120(7): 2011–6.
49. Alster TS, Tanzi EL. Laser surgery in dark skin. Skin Med 2003; 2: 80–5.
50. Tanzi EL, Alster TS. Cutaneous laser surgery in darker skin phototypes. Cutis 2004; 73: 21–30.
51. Ho C, Nguyen Q, Lowe NJ et al. Laser resurfacing in pigmented skin. Dermatol Surg 1995; 21: 1035–7.
52. Tanzi EL, Lupton JR, Alster TS. Review of lasers in dermatology: four decades of progress. J Am Acad Dermatol 2003; 49: 1–31.
53. Tanzi EL, Alster TS. Treatment of atrophic facial scars with a dual-mode erbium:YAG laser. Dermatol Surg 2002; 28: 551–5.
54. Sriprachya-Anunt S, Marchell NL, Fitzpatrick RE et al. Facial resurfacing in patients with Fitzpatrick skin type IV. Lasers Surg Med 2002; 30: 86–92.
55. Alster TS, Lupton JR. Prevention and treatment of side effects and complications of cutaneous laser resurfacing. Plast Reconstr Surg 2002; 109: 308–16.
56. Walia S, Alster TS. Prolonged clinical and histological effects from CO2 laser resurfacing of atrophic acne scars. Dermatol Surg 1999; 25: 926–30.
57. Tanzi EL, Alster TS. Side effects and complications of variable pulsed erbium:YAG laser skin resurfacing: extended experience with 50 patients. Plast Reconstr Surg 2003; 111: 1524–9.
58. Tanzi EL, Alster TS. Single-pass carbon dioxide versus multiple pass Er:YAG laser skin resurfacing: a comparison of postoperative wound healing and side effect rates. Dermatol Surg 2003; 29: 80–4.
59. Bhatt N, Alster TS. Laser surgery in dark skin. Dermatol Surg 2008; 34: 184–95.
60. Jeong JT, Kye YC. Resurfacing of pitted facial acne scars with a long-pulsed Er:YAG laser. Dermatol Surg 2001; 27(2): 107–10.
61. Alster TS. Preoperative patient considerations. In: Alster TS. Manual of cutaneous laser techniques, editor. 2nd ed. Philadelphia: Lippincott Williams & Wilkins, 2000: 13–32.
62. West TB, Alster TS. Effect of pretreatment on the incidence of hyperpigmentation following cutaneous CO2 laser resurfacing. Dermatol Surg 1999; 25: 15–7.
63. McDonald WS, Beasly D, Jones C. Retinoic acid and CO2 laser resurfacing. Plast Reconstr Surg 1999; 7: 2229–35.
64. Manstein D, Herron GS, Sink RK, Tanner H, Anderson RR. Fractional photothermolysis: a new concept for cutaneous remodeling using microscopic patterns of thermal injury. Lasers Surg Med 2004; 34: 426–38.
65. Hasegawa T, Matsukura T, Mizuno Y et al. Clinical trial of a laser device called fractional thermolysis system for acne scars. J Dermatol 2006; 33: 623–7.
66. Alster TS, Tanzi EL, Lazarus M. The use of fractional laser phothermolysis for the treatment of atrophic scars. Dermatol Surg 2007; 33: 295–9.
67. Patel N, Clement M. Selective nonablative treatment of acne scarring with 585 nm flashlamp pulsed dye laser. Dermatol Surg 2002; 28(10): 942–5.
68. Bjerring P, Clement M, Heickendorff L et al. Selective nonablative wrinkle reduction by laser. J Cutan Laser Ther 2000; 2: 9–15.
69. Keller R, Junior WB, Valente NYS, Rodrigues CJ. Nonablative 1,064-nm Nd:YAG laser for treating atrophic facial acne scars: histologic and clinical analysis. Dermatol Surg 2007; 33: 1470–6.
70. Wilkins JW, Voorhees JJ. Prevalence of nodulocystic acne in white and Negro males. Arch Dermatol 1970; 102: 631–4.
71. Kelly AP, Sampson DD. Recalcitrant nodulocystic acne in black Americans: treatment with isotretinoin. J Nat Med Assoc 1987; 79: 1266–70.
72. Fleischer AB Jr, Simpson JK, McMichael A, Feldman SR. Are there racial and sex differences in the use of oral isotretinoin for acne management in the United States? J Am Acad Dermatol 2003; 49(4): 662–6.
73. Perez A, Sanchez JL. Treatment of acne vulgaris in skin of color. Cosmetic Derm 2003; 16: 23–8.
74. American Academy of Dermatology. Pomade acne. [WWW document.] URL http://www.skincarephysicians.com/acnenet/pomadeacne.html (Accessed November 2008).

16 Treatment algorithm for acne scars
†*Daniele Innocenzi and Ilaria Proietti*

KEY FEATURES

Postacne scarring is a very distressing and difficult problem for physician and patient alike. The type of scarring following acne eruptions is also variable and often mixed. The most common permanent findings are diffused depressed scars. Other forms of irregularities include hypo–hyperpigmentation, hypertrophy, keloids, and cutaneous fistula.

To adequately address the patient with scarring, a true knowledge of the pathophysiology and anatomy of the different types of scars should be sought. Although this classic pathophysiology is shared, the subsequent evolution of the acne lesion and the degree of inflammation at clinical presentation may vary among individuals according to all skin phototypes. The morphology of each scar must be assessed and treatment designed accordingly.

Therapy needs to reflect patient characteristics such as age, gender, pubertal status, lifestyle, motivation, and coexisting conditions. Postacne scarring may be a psychologically devastating disease and degrades quality of life.

Recently, newer techniques and modifications to older ones may make this refractory problem more manageable. Options and treatment algorithm for dealing with postacne scarring are explored and a systematic review of literature is performed.

The wide variety of new treatment methods for postacne scarring includes the advent of tissue undermining, newer resurfacing tools, and possibly some future surgical and laser techniques.

One should attempt to match each scar against an available treatment as far as possible. Many of these techniques may be performed in a single treatment session, but multiple treatments are often necessary.

INTRODUCTION

Scarring occurs in all types of acne, not just in nodulocystic disease, but does vary with the severity and delay until effective treatment is organized. Some degree of postacne scarring is an outcome in 95% of patients with acne.(1) Postacne scarring can be particularly devastating and may even trigger suicidal ideation.(2) Interventions have to limit the disease, and thereby, its long-lasting fallout of both physical and emotional scars. Aggressive treatment of acne that is prone to scarring occasionally prevents this outcome.(3–5) Once scarring has occurred, patients and physicians are left to struggle with the options available for improving the appearance of the skin. Treating acne scars, according to Fulton, "is perhaps the most difficult cosmetic surgery procedure that exists."(6) It is really challenging to achieve total correction of tissue destruction caused by severe inflammatory acne, which can destroy the epidermis, dermis, and the underlying fat. The main treatment goal is to obtain as much improvement as possible rather than perfection.

DIFFUSION TREATMENTS

Acne vulgaris is a common disorder in people of all ethnic skin types. This ubiquitous disease of early and midlife occurs across the range of skin phototypes, from pale white to dark brown or black (95 to 100% of 16- to 17-year-old boys and 83% to 85% of 16- to 17-year-old girls).(7–10)

Acne has been shown to persist into adult life and a recent study of adults over 25 years of age revealed at least mild disease in 3% of men and 12% of women.(11) In recent years, the literature has begun to acknowledge that race and ethnicity are also parameters that need to be considered in acne management. The current (very limited) evidence base (12) indicates that there are probably no fundamental differences in acne epidemiology, pathophysiology (except for so called pomade acne in African American patients) (13), or basic treatment options across the spectrum of skin types. However, given the prevailing racial and ethnic disparities in access to healthcare (14), such survey results must be interpreted cautiously. Several key differences related to acne sequelae do stand out—especially the elevated risk of hyperpigmentation and keloids formation in those with darker skin.(15, 16) Clinicians need to be aware of these differences because they may require additions to the "standard" treatment algorithms to accommodate patients with darker skin. As the U.S. population of individuals with dark skin continues to increase (e.g., the proportion of the U.S. population that is White, non-Hispanic, is projected to decline steadily from 70% in 2003 to 50% in 2060) (17), these issues will soon spread beyond the domain of dermatologists specializing in ethnic skin to all dermatologists and primary care practitioners.

For most patients acne remains a nuisance with occasional flares of unsightly comedones, pustules, and nodules. For other less fortunate persons, the severe inflammatory response to *propionibacterium* acnes results in permanent disfiguring scars.(18) Acne scarring was recorded in 14% of women and 11% of men.(1)

HISTORY

As far back as 1905, surgical methods have been used to improve the skin that has been scarred by facial acne.(19) The work of the dermatologist Kromayer at the beginning of the 20th century (20–26) was instrumental in the development of dermabrasion, once the main treatment modality for skin resurfacing.

(27) Advances in equipment, techniques, and anesthesia have steadily occurred over the last three decades with wire brushes, diamond-embedded fraises, and serrated wheels being utilized. (28–34) In 1941, Eller and Wolff (35) first performed phenol peelings. Mechanisms used to resurface the epidermis and tighten the dermal collagen have included laser skin resurfacing CO (27, 36, 37) and Er:YAG (38) lasers or their combination. (39) Removal or leveling (or both) of individual scars has been achieved via excision, punch excision, punch elevation, dermal grafting, punch grafting, and subcision.(40–42)

Multiple other methods have been added to ablative techniques, including injections of collagen, (43) silicone (44) or fat (45), facelifts (46), and needling (47). Different authors have also tried to facilitate acne-scar treatment by suggesting schematic diagrams that correlate scars morphology and treatment, (48, 49) whereas others have used sequential therapeutic plans in treating theses scars.

Several excellent reviews of these scar revision modalities have been published.(50–54) However, according to the literature, the results of isolated ablative techniques are extremely variable, presenting effectiveness of outcomes that ranges from 25% to 81.4%.(55)

STRUCTURE AND FUNCTION AND DEVELOPMENTS IN PATHOPHYSIOLOGY

The first element in the evolution of an acne scar is evolution of acne itself. Acne vulgaris most commonly begins with a simple noninflammatory comedone of the pilosebaceous unit. In the lower part of the follicular wall, the horny cells become stickier, causing impaction of these horny cells and dilatation of the sebaceous follicle.(56)

Furthermore in comedonic skin condition *Propionibacterium acnes* flourishes and triggers production of the inflammatory stage of acne.

In uncomplicated cases, the comedone spontaneously uncaps to release the contained sebum and keratinous debris and may go on to develop into an inflamed acne lesion such as a papule, pustule, nodule, or cyst from, which likely leads to scarring.(Figure 16.1) A perifollicular abscess is due to ruptures through the weakened infrainfundibular section of the follicle. If the abscess rapidly encapsulates and communicates with the cornified layer, full release is still possible in 7 to 10 days with no sequelae.(57)

Scarring results when this process is incomplete or delayed. Failure to encapsulate results in further inflammatory progression and rupture. With this follicular explosion, hairs, lipids, keratin, free fatty acids, and released *Propionibacterium acnes* activate both classic and alternative complement pathways, amplifying the inflammation (58) in the dermis and leading to irritation in their new environment.(59) Thus, grouped open comedones or multichanneled fistulous tracts with interconnected keratinized tunnels may appear.(56) Prolonged inflammation of the follicular unit also promotes hyperplastic epithelialization, which is reflected clinically as ice-pick scars.(57)

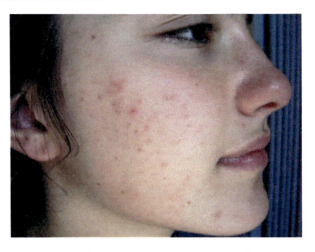

Figure 16.1 Grade I postacne scarring. A patient whose acne is coming under control with erythematous lesions treatment.

Other scars owe their appearance to the extent and the depth of the inflammation or perifollicular abscess formation that may directionally extend away from the cutaneous surface. If the dermal inflammation is severe and left untreated, sloughing is significant with total necrosis of the follicle, leading to severe dermal scarring as its sequela. Additional involvement of adjacent structures in the subcutis shows inflammatory migration along sweat glands and destruction of subcutaneous fat. When such deep inflammation occurs and transdermal abscess expulsion is not accomplished, nodules and cysts are the outcome.

Ongoing deep infection and inflammatory modulation of the pilosebaceous units often result in scarring that is either atrophic (Figure 16.2) or hyperplastic (hypertrophic or keloidal).(Figure 16.3–Figure 16.4) (60) As the scars mature, along with myoepithelial contraction caused by wound healing, they draw in the surface layers and cause atrophy, depressed craters, or indention. Much less commonly, acne scarring may become thickened (hypertrophic or keloidal) rather than atrophic. Certain individual characteristics seem to predispose patients to this type of acne scarring: These include family history, age between 10 and 30 years, and severity and site of inflammation. Keloid formation is also more common following acne in African-American, Hispanic, and Asian patients versus White patients. These keloidal overgrowths of scar tissue are seen between 5 and 16 times more frequently in patients with skin of color.(17)

If the acneiform activity is limited to the epidermis and superficial dermis, the disconcerting appearance may be only dyschromatic. It is common to observe immature processes as erythematous macules, especially within the first year of their onset. The return to normal pigmentation is often more prolonged in these lesions than other cutaneous trauma. Chronic macular inflammation may lead to permanent hypopigmentation or hyperpigmentation (especially seen in Fitzpatrick IV to VI skin types).(12)

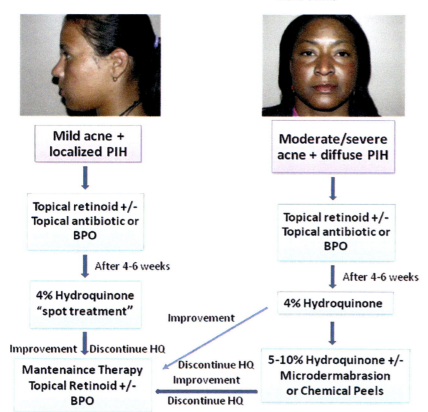

Figure 16.2 Trreatment algorithm for acne and post-inflammatory hyperpigmentation, adapted from Callender et al.

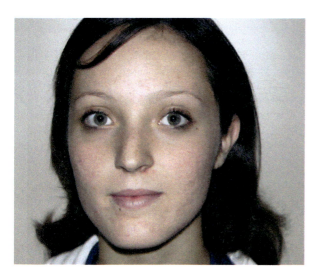

Figure 16.3 Grade II postacne scarring.

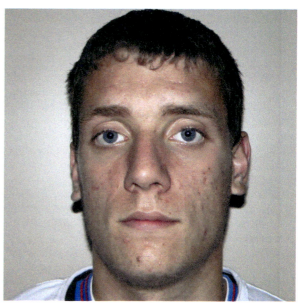

Figure 16.4 Grade III postacne scarring.

Table 16.1 Grades of Postacne Scarring.

Grade and Level	Characteristics
I. Macular	Erythematous, hyper- or hypo-pigmented flat marks visible to patient or observer at any distance
II. Mild	Mild atrophy or hypertrophy that may not be obvious at social distances of 50 cm or greater and may be covered adequately by makeup or the normal shadow of shaved beard hair in men or normal body hair if extrafacial
III. Moderate	Moderate atrophic or hypertrophic scarring that is obvious at social distances of 50 cm or greater and is not covered easily by makeup or the normal shadow of shaved beard hair in men or body hair if extrafacial, but is still able to be flattened by manual stretching of the skin (if atrophic)
IV. Severe	Severe atrophic or hypertrophic scarring that is obvious at social distances greater than 50 cm and is not covered easily by makeup or the normal shadow of shaved beard hair in men or body hair if extrafacial and is not able to be flattened by manual stretching of the skin

Table 16.2 Global Acne Scarring Classification: Types of Scars Making Up the Classification Grades.

Grade and Level	Examples of Scars
I. Macular	Erythematous, hyper- or hypo-pigmented flat marks
II. Mild	Mild rolling, small soft papular
III. Moderate	More significant rolling, shallow boxcar, mild-to-moderate hypertrophic or papular scars
IV. Severe	Punched-out atrophic (deep boxcar), ice-pick, bridges and tunnels, marked atrophy, dystrophic significant hypertrophy or keloid

Table 16.3 Global Acne-Scarring Classification and Likely Treatment Options.

Grade and Level	Examples of Scars
I. Macular	Time, optimized home skin care, light-strength peels, microdermabrasion, vascular or pigmented lasers, or intense pulsed light
II. Mild	Nonablative lasers, blood transfer, skin needling or rolling, microdermabrasion, dermal fillers
III. Moderate	Ablative lasers, dermabrasion, medical skin rolling, fractionated resurfacing, dermal fillers if focal, subcision and blood transfer. Intralesional corticosteroids steroids or fluorouracil and/or vascular laser if hypertrophic
IV. Severe	Punch techniques (float, excision grafting), focal trichloroacetic acid (CROSS technique) with or without resurfacing techniques (including fractionated resurfacing); fat transfer; occasionally rhytidectomy if grossly atrophic; intralesional corticosteroids steroids or fluorouracil and/or vascular laser if hypertrophic

TREATMENT

Therapeutic intervention for postacne scarring has historically been limited by the considerable morbidity of most treatments for only marginal disease improvement.(62)

Within the past decade, a requirement for developing successful treatments for postacne scarring is a greater understanding of its pathogenesis and variability of inflammatory mediators among afflicted individuals.(62)

New techniques have been added and older ones modified in attempts to improve risk–benefit profiles and less recuperation. One should assess both the overall appearance and the morphology of each scar and treatment designed accordingly. In literature authors have been using their own acne scar denominations and there are a lot of methods that encompass the majority of acne-scar types and correlate the lesions and the specific techniques used to repair them.(52, 55, 57)

To perform a treatment algorithm for dealing with postacne scarring we use the qualitative grading system of Goodman and Baron (Tables 16.1, 16.2, 16.3), which, in our opinion, is used as a template for describing the most suitable techniques to improve burden of disease of patients.(62)

MACULAR ACNE SCARRING AND MARKING (GRADE-1 ACNE SCARRING)

The first grade of scarring is macular changes of color and not of contour. Scars are visible irrespective of distance and may be red, white, or various shades of brown to black.(62)

ERYTHEMATOUS MACULES

Clinical aspects

If the scarring process is relatively superficial, only the epidermis and superficial dermis are involved. The scars may result as macules that may be erythematous if inflamed and comparatively early or young scars (under 1 year) or with altered pigmentation.(62) (**Figure 16.5**)

Often red macules improve over ensuing months spontaneously. Vascular laser therapy is useful for erythematous macules because red changes are quite well targeted by these light sources.(8) In theory, lasers may be useful to mature these scars more rapidly and useful for prevention of progression to scarring of inflamed healing-acne lesions.(63–65)

effectively (69–70), although their efficacy in the treatment of postinflammatory acne marking is not established.

Even if there is a risk of inducing postinflammatory hyperpigmentation with pigmented lesion lasers or light sources (71) such as neodymium-doped yttrium aluminium garnet (nd-YAG), Q-switching, intense pulsed light (IPL), these devices occasionally may be useful for resistant cases.(72)

HYPERPIGMENTED MACULES IN ETHNIC SKIN

Clinical aspects
Postinflammatory hyperpigmentation (PIH) presents clinically as hyperpigmented macules that correspond to the area of inflammation.(12) These lesions can be diffuse or localized and they can occur with or without secondary excoriation. The discoloration persists for months to years—much longer than the acne lesions themselves. For many patients, the lingering PIH is more psychologically disturbing than the original or residual acne itself.(12)

Treatment
In patients with darker skin early aggressive therapy for inflammatory acne combined with careful consideration of the patient's risk of irritation will help clinicians to eliminate PIH. Clinicians can achieve this balance in patients with ethnic skin with judicious use and prescription of widely available products. In addition, use of prevention strategies (e.g., sunscreen), special depigmenting agents (e.g., hydroquinone), and even adjunctive therapies (e.g., chemical peels or microdermabrasion) can be essential. According to Callender et al. we purpose the simplified algorithm in Figure 16.6.(12)

HYPOPIGMENTED MACULES

Clinical aspects
The white macules visible in the postacne scarring may be true scars or postinflammatory leukoderma.(62)

Treatment
Treatment of these lesions are very difficult and it is often without significant outcomes. In literature there is the description of an 11-year-old White female patient who was successfully treated with manual dermabrasion for a hypochromic scar on the left forearm.(73) Reports of improvement of these lesions by needle dermabrasion utilizing a tattoo gun without pigment (74) and pigment transfer procedures have been attempted.

Hypopigmented macular scarring also called perifollicular scarring have been reasonably refractory to treatment.

Perifollicular acne inflammation may result small hypopigmented macular scars from destruction of dermal components around the hair follicles and they are largely untreatable at the present time.(74)

Minigrafting also utilized for treatment of vitiligo, holds some promise in the treatment of postacne scarring.(75, 76) The most known epidermal suspensions are cultured for 24 hours, but an automated commercial kit for trypsin dermal

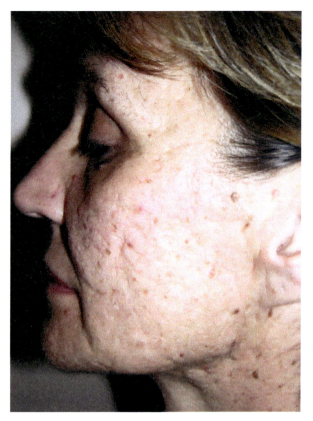

Figure 16.5 Grade IV postacne scarring.

Patients affected by *acne excoriée* with erythematous macules were been treated with psychotherapy and these kind of lasers (nd- YAG, Er:YAG, diode, IPL) with success.(66)

HYPERPIGMENTED MACULES

Clinical aspects
Pigmentation of scars may be increased in more olive-skinned patients and represents mostly a postinflammatory response that will fade in 3 to 18 months.(62)

Treatment
These scars need strict sun protection to guard against aggravating the hyperpigmentation, but barring sun protection requirement, further reparative treatment is not usually required. If patients seek treatment, medical therapy with topical reparative creams such retinol (vitamin A), tretinoin (retinoic acid) or hydroxyacids in conjunction with topical corticosteroids, hydroquinone, kojic acid, and azelaic acid used in other examples of postinflammatory pigmentation may be useful.(67–68) Alternatively or additionally low-strenght skin peels with glycolic and retinoic acids and Jessner's solution or its variants may also be utilized

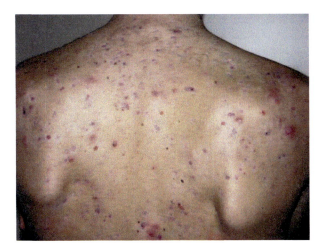

Figure 16.6 Inflammatory lesions and atrophic scars co-exist in the same patient.

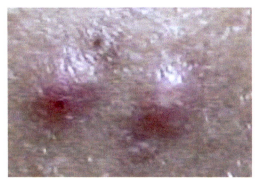

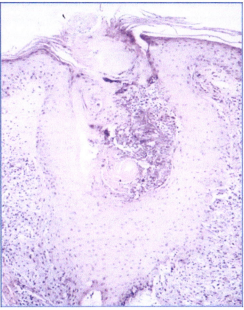

epidermal separation may improve the ease of the technique of minigrafting and allow immediately available, autologous, noncultured epidermal suspension (Re-Cell, Clinical Cell Culture Americas, Coral Springs, FL). This is now the most effective method.(77, 78)

MILD ATROPHY (GRADE 2 ACNE SCARRING)

Clinical aspects
This grade of scarring includes those scars that may not be obvious at social distances of 50 cm or greater and may be covered adequately by makeup or the normal shadow of shaved beard hair in men or normal body hair if extrafacial.(62) (Figure 16.7)

This equates to a superficial type of atrophic scar or **mild rolling scar**. Mild rolling scars are usually wider than 4 to 5 mm and have abnormal fibrous anchoring of the dermis. to the subcutis. Correction of the subdermal component is essential for treatment success.(62)

TREATMENT OF PATIENTS WITH FEW SCARS

Tissue Augmentation
The group with few scars benefits from fairly simple treatments. The past decade has seen the advent of many nonautologous biologic and nonbiologic tissue augmentation agents that may be used for atrophic scar contour correction. Achievement of safe, long-term or permanent correction using a tissue augmentation agent is a burgeoning area of interest.(79)

The short-term correction agents that are in use include injectable fillers, including bovine, human, or swine collagen; polylactic acid; and hyaluronic or agarose acid. Usually 2 or 3 treatment sessions are required for the best possible skin correction, which may need time in the range of 6 months to 1 or 2 years for correction to be attained.

Figure 16.7a Clinical and histological features of inflamed acne lesions.

I phase (**6–24 hours**)
Increase of neutrophilic cells into follicle (suppurative folliculitis) and of lymphocytes around pilosebaceus unit (perifolliculitis)

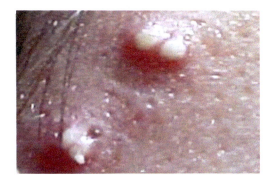

Figure 16.7b Grade 3 acne scarring.

Silicon variations of polyacrylamides and expanded polytetrafluoroethylene are agents used for longer correction.(80) There are not sufficiently accurate for improvement of mild scarring due to important local immunologic events.

However, all dermal augmentation agents may cause immunomediated adverse events or simply not be perfectly placed.(80)

Goodman et al. (81) described hematogenous transfer for tissue augmentation by the use of the patient's whole blood. This agent was investigated for its ability to present an exogenous chromophore that can be used by monochromatic laser or polychromatic light as a suitable target.

Blood is injected immediately after drawing by simple injection with a 1-mL syringe with attached 30-gauge needle high up in the dermis distending the scar giving a bleb with a bruised appearance. This treatment may be repeated at monthly intervals until adequate improvment is attained. Excessive fluence may be counterproductive because further collagen deposition is to induced by a low-level heat injury.(26, 27)

TREATMENT OF PATIENTS WITH MANY SCARS

Microdermabrasion
Dermabrasion was the first resurfacing technique that aided patients with this disorder.(1) Over the last three decades we have observed advances in techniques, equipment, and anesthesia and the exceeding of the manual dermoabrasion.

New handpieces with 20,000 to 30,000 rpm have helped to control the depth of injury and reproducibility of treatment. Performed on frozen or tumesced facial skin, dermabrasion removes tissue to the level of the papillary dermis, or in significant scarring, the upper reticular dermis.(57)

Microdermabrasion using aluminum oxide crystals has attracted some considerable attention for acne scarring.(82) Small crystals of aluminium oxide are fired against the skin from a nozzle housing a compression and aspiration system; this causes multiple small lacerations, and used crystals are aspirated back from the skin surface and discarded. Multiple treatments are required.(57)

Before starting any resurfacing procedure, it is exceptionally important to discuss with the patient the possible outcomes, including nature of healing, postsurgical care, and potential complications. Specific inquiries about infectious conditions, prior herpetic outbreaks, keloid formation, bleeding diathesis, and prior isotretinoin treatment are required.(83)

Even if dermabrasion as a procedure is risk prone and may lead to scarring and dyschromia and results point to substantial variation in clinical outcomes, it is indeed a low-cost alternative to laser therapy and forms an integral part of the armamentarium of the practitioner involved in the treatment of acne scarring.(28, 32, 33)

Skin Needling
Skin needling is an effective method for treating acne scars because it involves puncturing the skin multiple times with a small needle to induce collagen growth. Since 1995 Orentreich and Orentreich (42) have used this tecnique to achieve percutaneous collagen induction (PCI). Desmond Fernandes (47), simultaneously and independently, used skin needling to treat the upper lip by inserting a 15-gauge needle into the skin and then tunneling under the wrinkles in various directions. Camirand and Doucet (49) treated scars with a tattoo gun to "needle abrade" them.(74) Although this technique could be used on many areas, it was laboriously slow and the holes in the epidermis were too close and too shallow. All these techniques worked because the needles break old collagen strands in the most superficial layer of the dermis that tether scars or wrinkles. It is presumed that this process promotes removal of damaged collagen growth and induces more collagen immediately under the epidermis.

A special new device covered with 30-gauge needles (Dermaroller TM) is now available. It may be rolled horizontally, vertically, and diagonally, right and left, over the areas affected by acne scars. The microneedles penetrate through the epidermis and for about 1.5 to 2 mm into the dermis. The epidermis is only punctured and rapidly heals. After the treatment, the skin bleed for a short time. When bleeding stops, the serous ooze formed may be removed from the surface of the skin with using sterile saline solution. After each session of treatment, patients' facial skin appears reddened and swollen but redness and swelling disappear in 2 to 3 days. No side effect was described or found and every area of the face and the body maybe treated.(84)

With this technique the rolling is continued and done once in a month until some bruising is noted.

The mechanism of action of the collagen induction therapy (CIT) is based on scientific facts that skin cells communicate by electrical signals. When the skin is microneedled, cells react to this intrusion by changing their internal electrical potential. This electrical charge in return stimulates skin cells to release chemical compositions, protein, and growth factors. Proliferated skin cells, such as fibroblasts, migrate to the point of injury and transform into collagen fibers.(50)

CIT is a simple technique and can have an "immediate effect" on the improvement of rolling acne scars. In accordance with the literature, a complete result after CIT may be observed after 8 to 12 months of treatment as the deposition of new collagen takes place slowly. Compared with other ablative methods, CIT has advantages. The most important one is that the epidermis remains intact because it is not damaged, eliminating most of the risks and negative side effects of chemical peeling, laser resurfacing, or dermoabrasion.

This treatment appears to be synergistic with other methods such as nonablative lasers, blood transfer, and vascular lasers. Goodman et al. (62) suggest to always supplement the procedure of skin rolling with other procedures, both simultaneously (blood transfer, vascular laser, and subcision for bigger scars) and sequentially starting 1 month after the procedure and continuing monthly for 3 treatments (nonablative 1,450-nm diode laser).

A recently introduced laser employing the concept of "fractionated photothermolysis" produces small, vertical zones of full-thickness thermal damage by a midinfrared laser.(85) This is a method of ablative resurfacing without a pronounced and long healing phase and conceptually it may be the laser equivalent of skin needling.

Nonablative Lasers. Laser skin resurfacing has become a popular therapeutic modality for the correction of acne scars, but it is not always effective in all types of acne scars. Nonablative dermal remodelling has gained acceptance in the treatment of atrophic scars and to have a role especially in rolling and shallow boxcar scars respect to ice-pick and deep boxcar scars.(86)

Although improvement is seen with nonablative lasers, most investigators conclude that the results do not approach those of ablative lasers requiring subsequent reepithelialization. For the patient, the trade-off is between less improvement and more recovery time, as a longer recovery time is necessary to ensure proper healing.

The major lasers used for this purpose are the midinfrared lasers as diode,short-pulsed, variable-pulsed, and dual-mode Er:YAG, Nd:YAG lasers, and fractionated photothermolysis. (86, 87)

As opposed to laser resurfacing using CO^2 these lasers minimize epidermal damage by cooling the epidermis while targeting water within the dermis as its active chromophore produce a diffuse dermal injury heating to above 501C.(86–90) As a result, reepithelialization is avoided during the recovery period. In addition, new models in this area have further reduced epidermal injury by cooling the skin with a cryogen spray (CoolTouch, Laser Aesthetics) to maintain an epidermal temperature between 42 and 481C.(82)

Repeated treatments are required with a suitably higher benefit–risk ratio, but longevity of result is still largely unknown.

Much speculation surrounds the mechanisms by which nonablative dermal remodeling occurs, (91) despite its documented clinical and histologic efficacy in the treatment of rhytides.(92–94) Recently, the concept of a beneficial subclinical epidermal injury has been raised with nonablative laser resurfacing.(95) Such superficial dermal blood vessel injury and cytokine release, with potentially enhanced dermal remodeling, could explain the results.

Subcision techniques or skin needling in conjunction with nonablative lasers may be used in patients presenting milder to slightly more severe scarring.

MODERATE ATROPHY (GRADE 3 DISEASE)

Clinical aspects
This level of scarring is obvious at social distances of 50 cm or greater and is not covered easily by makeup or the normal shadow of shaved beard hair in men or body hair if extrafacial, but is still able to be flattened by manual stretching of the skin (Table 16.1).(62) **Figure 16.8**.

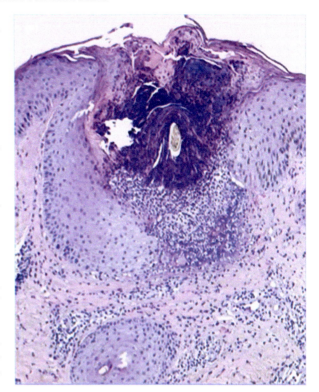

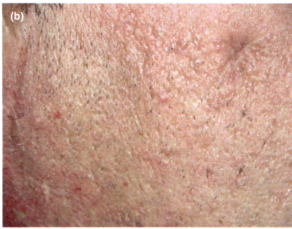

Figure 16.8 (a) II phase (**48 hours**) Ruptures through the weakened infrainfundibular section of the follicle cause perifollicular abscess. (suppurative perifolliculitis). (b) Clinical aspect of atrophic scars.

It equates to the **deep rolling** and **shallow boxcar atrophic-type scars**.

Shallow (0.1–0.5 mm) boxcar atrophic-type scars are round to oval depressions with sharply demarcated vertical edges, similar to varicella scars. They are clinically wider at the surface than ice-pick scars and do not taper to a point at the base.(62)

TREATMENT OF PATIENTS WITH FEW SCARS

If there are few scars then their augmentation by temporary or longer-term autologous or external agents may be appropriate. Combinations of techniques such as subcision, blood transfer, nonablative or vascular laser, and skin needling may be useful for more significant scarring.

Subcision. The technique of subcutaneous incision, or Subcision, was initially described by Orentreich and Orentreich (42) in 1995. It is used to free the tethering fibrous bands that cause deep rolling and shallow boxcar atrophic-type scars.

For this procedure, the entire area to be subcised is marked and subcutaneous anesthetic is administered. A hypodermic needle may be used (18–26 gauge depending on scar size and depth) to cut the adherent bands beneath the skin. Excellent results can be achieved by using an 18-gauge, 1½-inch NoKor Admix needle (Becton Dickinson and Co, Franklin Lakes, NJ). The triangular tip (similar to a No. 11 blade) allows smooth and thorough separation of the fibrous cords.(43, 44) The actions consist in tunneling parallel to the skin surface using a gentle pistonlike motion to advance the needle through the fibrous bands in order to release epidermis from upper dermis.(42)

This process leads to a pooling of blood under the defect keeping the scar base from immediately reattaching to the surface layers. Blood accumulates under the defect, and its subsequent organization is thought to result in connective tissue formation. Most atrophic acne scars improve well with 1 to 3 treatments. This technique may be readily combined with resurfacing and this leads to long-term correction of the defect.

The technique of undermining scars has been practiced as an adjunct to fibrin foam or collagen implantation, dermal grafting, and microlipoinjection.(79, 80)

Risks of subcision include bleeding (which is uncommon with proper anesthesia and pressure bandages) and excessive fibroplasia leading to nodule formation. This rare outcome can be improved with low-dose intralesional steroid injections, but often resolves without treatment in 2 to 3 months. Bruising from the procedure fades within 1 to 2 week.

As a simple technique that appears to produce long-term correction of contour defects, it deserves to be a first-line treatment for many isolated moderate atrophic scars.(79)

TREATMENT OF PATIENTS WITH MANY SCARS

Technique-sensitive Resurfacing (lasers, radiofrequency, medium-strength peels, plasma, and abrasion).

The atrophic forms in this group are improved by ablative laser resurfacing if widespread atrophy is seen. CO_2 laser was the laser system first utilized for postacne scarring (39), commonly replacing dermabrasion (drywall/plaster-sanding screen (96) or moistened silicone carbide sandpaper (97)) and strong chemical peeling (98). These newer adaptations of older techniques still suffer from a prolonged healing phase and morbidity. Although other lasers have been added to the armamentarium, it is uncertain whether they add much to the efficacy.(99) Modulating the erbium laser has meant that it behaves more like a CO_2 laser with arguably a better safety profile.(89) Another popular method has been to combine erbium and CO_2 lasers either simultaneously or sequentially. (100, 101)The statements made above regarding the excessive morbidity of resurfacing techniques, however, are almost as true for these newer lasers.(102–104) The greatest fear for those performing laser resurfacing is the incidence of hypopigmentation. The use of trypsin-digested donor epidermal cells after the resurfacing may allow a protection from this complication and a more rapid epithelialization. In an effort to increase penetration depth and strive toward collagen shrinkage and skin tightening, radiofrequency wavelengths have been extensively employed.(105) Radiofrequency devices produce electrical energy that heats the dermis without plume and at relatively low temperatures. The first energy source in this arena was the monopolar radiofrequency device, ThermaCool (Thermage, Inc, Hayward, Calif), which demonstrated improvement in skin laxity and acne scars. The most recent development is the Accent device (Alma Lasers, Ltd, Caesarea, Israel), which offers alternatively bipolar and a novel unipolar RF modes.(106–110)The treatment of photoaging through nonablative photorejuvenation encompasses the use of PDT.(111) The application of topical photosensitizers, namely, 5-ALA, for short incubation times combined with newer laser and light sources has been shown to be safe and effective. It may have a role in the collagen growth and thus in improvement of atrophic scars.

This may also benefit from the treatments described in the milder group, especially medical skin rolling combined simultaneously with subcision and later by nonablative laser. (111)

SEVERE ATROPHY (GRADE 4 ACNE SCARRING)

Clinical aspects

This is represented by severe atrophic scarring that is obvious at social distances of 50 cm or greater and is not covered easily by makeup or the normal shadow of shaved beard hair in men or body hair if extrafacial and is not able to be flattened by manual stretching of the skin (Table 16.1).(64) **Figure 16.9– Figure 16.10**

ICE-PICK SCARS

Deep ice-pick scars are narrow (<2 mm) and fibrotic scars, with sharp shoulders perpendicular to the skin. They are epithelial invaginations that can reach the subcutaneous layer. The surface opening is usually, but not always, wider than the deeper infundibulum as the scar tapers from the surface to its deepest apex.

PUNCHED-OUT ATROPHIC

Punched-out atrophic or deep boxcar scars are depressions (≥0.5 mm) with sharply demarcated, vertical edges (1.5 to 4.0 mm).

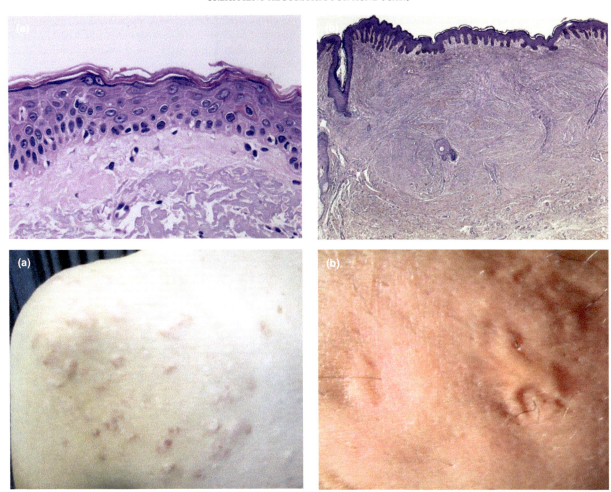

Figure 16.9 Clinical and histological features of hypertrophic scars.

Figure 16.10 Clinical and histological features of keloyd.

Tunnels are constituted of two or more ice picks connected by an epithelized tract. They have to be excised but can also be repaired by punch grafting.(112)

Dystrophic scars. These types of scars may have irregular or star-like shapes with a white and atrophic floor. They can also be represented by fibrotic masses with multichanneled tracts that retain sebaceous or pustular material.

MARKED ATROPHY

Marked atrophy is a deficit seen in patients with acne were disrupted acne follicles and cysts release inflammatory mediators that destroy facial fat. Cysts are also space-occupying lesions that leave avoid after their resolution that the atrophied subcutaneous tissues cannot fill.

Aging exaggerates this lipoatrophy and the concavities of the preauricular, temples, inframalar, and perioral tissues become exaggerated and scarring in these regions appears worse.

Treatment
Larger punched-out scars (deep boxcar and larger ice-pick scars) have to be excised by cylindrical punches (113), which have to be large enough to involve the entire lesion and by elevation or float techniques. They can be left to second intention healing or be replaced by full-thickness grafts from the postauricular area, which are 25% to 50% larger than the defect (punch-graft technique).(51, 55, 113) Direct closure of these small holes very frequently leads to enlarged and unpleasant scars, unless they are submitted to deep intradermal. More recently, the use of focal trichloroacetic acid at high concentrations (60%–100 %, CROSS technique) (114), especially in the treatment of smaller ice-pick and poral-type scars, has always been difficult. This technique requires multiple sessions until the center of the scar is seen to flatten, basically scarring the inside of the cylindrical scar, making it cosmetically more appealing.

119

Dystrophic scars are treated by direct excision under primary elliptical or broken lines, and sometimes even "M", "Z", or "W" plasties are required for their treatment.(46, 55)

In the treatment of marked atrophy, fat is an excellent deeper augmentation material because it is cheap and readily avaible. This technique is also termed lipofilling, which does not result in rejectction or allergic reactions. Fat is probably a permanent augmentation technique (more than 50% of transplanted fat survives) (115, 116), and correctly implanted, it produces accurate, longstanding, and autologous correction.(117–119) It is useful to combine this augmentation with most other surface techniques such as resurfacing or subcision. Fat is injected through a small nick made with a vented needle (Nokor, Becton Dickinson), 11-gauge blade, or similar instrument. To achieve precision of correction, undermining or subcision (42) is used to release the scar tissue from its attachments to deeper tissues. The residual fat may always be frozen and may be used for at least 12 months after the procedure.

Most acne-scarred patients benefit from further top-up procedures 3 months after the procedure. Overcorrection should be kept to no more than 10%. Aging adds to the problems of the acne-scarred face and influences patients to seek corrective surgery. Polylactic acid and hyaluronic acid may be used to augment substantially depressed acne scarring if fat is not available.

MILD, MODERATE, AND SEVERE HYPERTROPHIC DISEASE

Clinical aspects
Much less commonly, though, acne scarring may become thickened (papular, bridges, hypertrophic, keloids scars) rather than becoming atrophic. Certain individual characteristics seem to predispose patients to this type of acne scarring.

Papular scars. Papular scars may be small, soft, papular (Grade 2 Mild) or more significant papular scars (Grade 3 Moderate). Papules are soft elevations, like anetodermas, which are frequently observed on the trunk and chin area.(62)

Treatment
They are largely untreatable at the present time, but if scars are facial, they can be treated by controlled CO_2 laser vaporization or light electrodesiccation of each papule.(55)

Bridges. Bridge, another kind of elevated scar, is a fibrous string over healthy skin (Grade 4 Severe). This type of scars is common on the face.

Treatment
They are treated by tangential excision.(61)

HYPERTROPHIC AND KELOIDS SCARS
Hypertrophic scars are also thickened elevations, but remain within the confines of the original acne lesion with the scar progressing for a few months and then slowing before regressing after some years.

Histologically, hypertrophic scars show numerous fibroblasts but relatively few collagen bundles, but with some myofibroblasts, and this may explain the scar contracture that is seen. (Grade 4 Severe)

Keloids scars spread outside the confines of the original wound. They have differences in fibroblast size and activity, immune cell actions, and an imbalance between production and degradation of excess collagen. They are common in the mandibular arch, shoulders, and sternal region and are prone to recur.(61, 62) (Grade 4 Severe)

Treatment

Topical silicone-gel sheeting
Topical silicone-gel sheeting alone or with intralesional steroids are the only evidence-based, recommendable forms of treatment to control the quality of a scar. The advantages and disadvantages of both are well known. Signorini et al. (120) first verified the efficacy of a new topical self-drying spreadable silicone gel (Dermatix®, Valeant Pharmaceuticals, Milan, Italy) in a prospective trial involving a group of 160 patients. Considering the effective results obtained and the good patient compliance, the authors rated this concept of treatment as the first choice for preventing hypertrophy of recent scars (such as hypertrophic and keloidal postacne scarring). This report was also confirmed by other authors later.(121–125)

INTRALESIONAL CYTOTOXIC THERAPY
The use of corticosteroid injections, to date, is the core treatment available for the management of excessive tissue production in scars. Currently, the most effective and safe regimen for hypertrophic and keloidal acne management appears to be the use of corticotherapy injection of intradermal steroids (triamcinolone acetonide 10 or 40 mg/ml or betamethasone sodium phosphate and betamethasone acetate 5.7 mg/ml). (126) Usually it is best to start with triamcinolone acetonide (10 mg/ml) or betamethasone sodium phosphate and betamethasone acetate (5.7 mg/ml), reserving triamcinolone acetonide (40 mg/ml) for resistant cases.

There has also been recent interest in the intralesional use of the cytotoxics fluorouracil and bleomycin sulphate, however, (127, 128) as treatments of these lesions. Fluorouracil is usually utilized at a concentration of 50 mg/mL and has been mixed 80:20 with low-strength intralesional steroid. It may be used alone, however. Usually approximately 1 mL is utilized in each session and often 0.1 to 0.3 mL is all that is required for an individual scar. Recently the molecular basis of the action of fluorouracil has been elucidated. Fluorouracil appears to be a potent inhibitor of TGF-b/SMAD signalling.(129)

VASCULAR LASERS
Alster TS et al. first reported treatment of keloid sternotomy scars with 585 nm flashlamp-pumped pulsed-dye laser with improvement in scar height, skin texture, erythema, and pruritus in the

laser-treated scars.(130) This work of 1995 has been confirmed by more recent studies.(131, 132)

OTHER THERAPIES

Rusciani et al. treated 135 patients to assess the efficacy of cryotherapy in the treatment of keloids with good results. The main adverse effects reported were atrophic depressed scars and residual hypopigmentation but no recurrences arose during the follow-up period.(133) It is useful to combine cryotherapy with other modalities such as surgery or corticosteroids.

Other authors described surgical excision and immediate postoperative adjuvant irradiation with X or b radiotherapy (134, 135) More recently intralesional verapamil at a concentration of 2.5 mg/mL (0.5–2 mL injected volume depending on the size of the scar) (136) or topical imiquimod (137) have been suggested as postoperative adjunctive treatment to surgical excision of keloidal.

OUTLOOK—FUTURE DEVELOPMENTS

In clinical practice, it is common to observe some patients with inflammatory acne suffer from significant scarring, while others with apparently similar severity are able to heal without scarring. It is known that there are both humoral and cellular-immune components that correlate with the severity of acne and that antigens of *Propionibacterium* acnes play a central role and the extent of this response has been found to differ among patients.(138)

Holland et al. (138) examined this by assessing whether there were differences in the cell-mediated immune responses at different time points in inflamed lesion development between resolution in patients who were prone and those with the same degree of inflamed acne but who were not prone to develop scarring.

In lesions of nonscarring patients, the time course was typical of a type-IV, delayed-hypersensitivity response, a significant angiogenesis with preferential recruitment of macrophages and Langerhans cells with high cellular HLA-DR expression that indicates the clearance of causal antigen(s).

In addition, these patients are not highly sensitized to the antigen(s) responsible for acne because they have CD4+ T cells, with an even smaller number being specifically skin homing.

Thus, there is effective removal of the causal antigen(s) and the satisfactory resolution of the inflammatory.

In lesions from patients who scar, the scenario was different. In early lesions, they have a low cellular HLA-DR expression and an ineffectual early inflammatory response.

In resolving lesions, the number of CD4+ T cells in the infiltrate and angiogenesis remained high and these would lead to abnormal healing and pathological scarring in these patients.

Thus, based on the poorly resolving inflammation, scarring would be a more likely outcome, suggesting the requirement of antiinflammatory medications.

In addition, prolonged angiogenesis may play an important role in the developing of postacne atrophic scars. Blood vessels to cut a path and invade into subcutaneous layer require increase in metalloproteinases. The matrix metalloproteinases

(MMPs) are a family of zinc metallo endopeptidases (MMP 1F Type 1 collagenase, MMP 2F Type 4 collagenase, and MMP 3F stromelysin-1) that can collectively cleave all components of the extracellular matrix and allow vascular proliferation.(139–142) Healing induces many changes to the collagen content of the wound; both the collagen type and positioning of the fibers are altered as the scar tissue develops. Tissue inhibitors of metalloproteinases (TIMPs) control their activity because if metalloproteinases are overactive or active for a longer time than required to support prolonged angiogenesis, the dissolution of dermal support or a breakdown of the normal balance of collagen production may occur.

So if we are to intervene with physical therapies, it may seem reasonable to target poorly resolving angiogenesis also, and keeping this in mind, vascular lasers and light sources could be examined for possible treatment options. Common agents such as retinoic acid, imiquimod, calcipotriol, corticosteroids, low-dose fluorouracil, diclofenac, tetracyclines, hyaluronic acid, estrogen, metabolites, genestein, heparin, cyclosporine A, steroids, and COX2 inhibitors have all been suggested to be antiangiogenesis substances. Many of these agents have both antiinflammatory and antiangiogenesis characteristics and may deserve investigation to help avert early acne scarring.(143)

SUMMARY FOR CLINICIAN

Acne often results in secondary damage in the form of scarring. Even with prevention and good efforts, scars may occur. The aim of this work is to give a broad overview of multiple management options, whether medically, surgically, or procedurally based. It is also important to ensure that the patient is able to comply with therapy, and clear guidelines regarding treatment, possible adverse effects, and realistic expectations are to be provided before commencing therapy.

Levels of Evidence

Medical Management	Literature	Level of Evidence
Retinoids	Schmidt JB et al. 1999	2
Topical/injectable steroids	Berman B et al 2008	2
Silicone dressing	Signorini M et al. 2007	2
Various other topical or injectable substances	Copcu E et al. 2004	2
	Zeichner JA et al.2008	1

Surgical Management	Literature	Level of Evidence
Punch excision	Whang KK et al. 1999	2
Punch elevation	Arouete J et al. 1976	2
Skin graft	Alster TS et al. 1997	3
'Subcision'	Orentreich DS et al. 2005	2
Debulking	Kadunc BV et al. 2003	1

Procedural Management	Literature	Level of Evidence
Cryosurgery	Rusciani L et al. 2006	2
Elettrodessication	Doornbos JF et al. 1990	3
Radiation treatment	Akita S et al. 2007	2
	Arons JA et al. 2008	3
Chemical peels	Landau M et al. 2005	2
	Lee JB et al. 2002	2
Microdermabrasion	Zisser M et al. 1995	3
	Savardekar P. et al. 2007	3
Dermabrasion	Goodman GJ 1994	2
	Alt T et al. 1997	2
Needling	Fabbrocini G et al. (in press)	2
	Fernandes D et al. 2005	2

Tissue Augmentation	Literature	Level of Evidence
Autografts	Pinski KS 1992	2

Ablative Lasers	Literature	Level of Evidence
CO$_2$ laser	Walia S et al. 1999	2
Erbium:yttrium-garnet Nd-Yag	Woo SH et al. 1994	1
Fractionated laser	Alster TS et al. 2007	2

Non Ablative Lasers	Literature	Level of Evidence
532-nm KTP laser	Baugh WP et al. 2005	1
510/585-nm Pulsed dye	Alster TS et al. 1993	1
1064/1320-nm Nd-Yag	Lipper GM et al. 2006	2
1450-nm Diode	Uebelhoer NS et al. 2007	3
1540 Er:glass	Fournier N et al. 2005	2

Light and Energy	Literature	Level of Evidence
Intense pulsed light	Bellew SG et al. 2005	2
Radiofrequency	Alster TS et al. 2007	2
Plasma	Bogle AB et al. 2007	3
	Potter MJ et al. 2007	3
Photodynamic therapy	Alexiades-Armenakas MR 2006	2

REFERENCES

1. Kromayer E. Kosmetische resultate bei anwedung des stanverfahrens. Dermatol Wochenschr 1935; 101: 1306.
2. Cotterill JA, Cunliffe WJ. Suicide in dermatological patients. Br J Dermatol 1997; 137: 246–50.
3. Barankin B, DeKoven J. Psychosocial effect of common skin diseases. Can Fam Physician 2002; 48: 712–6.
4. Mallon E, Newton JN, Klassen A et al. The quality of life in acne: a comparison with general medical conditions using generic questionnaires. Br J Dermatol 1999; 140: 672–6.
5. Kellett SC, Gawkrodger DJ. The psychological and emotional impact of acne and the effect of treatment with isotretinoin. Br J Dermatol 1999; 140: 273–82.
6. Fulton JE. Dermabrasion, chemabrasion and laser abrasion. Dermatol Surg 1996; 22: 619–28.
7. Burton JL, Cunliffe WJ, Stafford I et al. The prevalence of acne vulgaris in adolescence. Br J Dermatol 1971; 85: 119–26.
8. Munro-Ashman D. Acne vulgaris in a public school. Trans St John's Hosp Dermatol Soc 1963; 49: 144–8.
9. Rademaker M, Garioch JJ, Simpson NB. Acne in schoolchildren: no longer a concern for dermatologists. BMJ 1989; 298: 1217–9.
10. Bloch B. Metabolism, endocrine glands and skin disease, with special reference to acne vulgaris and xanthoma. Br J Dermatol 1931; 43: 61–87.
11. Goulden V, Stables GI, Cunliffe WJ. Prevalence of facial acne in adults. J Am Acad Dermatol 1999; 41: 577–80.
12. Callender VD. Acne in ethnic skin: special considerations for therapy. Dermatol Ther 2004; 17(2): 184–95.
13. Plewig G, Fulton JE, Kligman AM. Pomade acne. Arch Derm 1970; 101(5): 580–4.
14. Institute of Medicine. Unequal treatment: confronting racial and ethnic disparities in healthcare. Summary. Washington, DC: National Academies of Sciences, 2003.
15. Grimes PR, Stockton T. Pigmentary disorders in blacks. Dermatol Clin 1988; 6: 271–81.
16. Kelly AP. Keloids: pathogenesis and treatment. Cosmetic Derm 2003; 16: 29–32.
17. US Census Bureau. Population Projections Program, Washington D.C. Table NP-T5-B (middle series projections). January 13, 2000.
18. Leeming JP, Holland KT, Cunliffe WJ. The pathological and ecological significance of micro-organisms colonizing acne vulgaris comedones. J Med Microbiol 1985; 20: 11–6.
19. Kromayer E. Die Heilung der Akne durch ein neues narbenloses Operationverfahren. Munchen Med Wochenschr 1905; 52: 943.
20. Kromayer E. Rotationsinstrurnente. Ein neues technisches. Veffahren in der dermatologischen Kieinchirurgie. Dermatol Z 1995; 12: 26.
21. Kromayer E. Die Heilung der Akne durch ein neues narbenloses. Operationsverfahren: Das Stanzen. Illustr Monatsschr Aerztl Polytech 1905; 27: 101.

22. Kromayer E. Die Heilung der Akne durch ein neues narbenloses Operationsverfahren: Das Stanzen. Munch Med Wochenschr 1905; 52: 942.

23. Kromayer E. Eine neues sichere Epitationsmethode: Das Stanzen. Deutsche Med Wochenschr 1905; 31: 179.

24. Kromayer E. Cosmetic treatment of skin complaints. English translation of the second German edition (1929). New York: Oxford University Press, 1930: 9.

25. Kromayer E. Das Frasen in der Kosmetik. Kosmetalogische Rundschau 1933; 4: 61.

26. Kurtin A. Corrective surgical planning of the skin. Arch Dermatol Syph 1953; 68: 389–97.

27. Aronsson A, Erifsson T, Jacobsson S et al. Effects of dermabrasion on acne scarring: a review and a study of 25 cases. Acta Derm Venereol 1997; 77: 39–42.

28. LeVan P. Mechanical method of freezing the skin for surgical planing. Arch Dermatol Syph 1954; 69: 739–41.

29. Burks J. In: Dermabrasion and chemical peeling. Springfield (Ill): Charles C Thomas, 1979.

30. Yarborough J, Alt T. Current concepts in dermabrasion. J Dermatol Surg Oncol 1987; 13: 595–6.

31. Alt T. Facial dermabrasion: advantages of the diamond fraise technique. J Dermatol Surg Oncol 1987; 13: 618–24.

32. Alt TH, Goodman, GJ, Coleman III WP et al. Dermabrasion. In: Coleman WP, Hanke CW, Alt TH, et al. eds. Cosmetic surgery of the skin. 2nd ed. St. Louis: Mosby-Year Book Inc., 1997: 112–51.

33. Goodman GJ, Richards S. The treatment of facial wrinkles and scars. Mod Med 1994; 37: 50–63.

34. Goodman GJ. Dermabrasion using tumescent anaesthesia. J Dermatol Surg Oncol 1994; 20: 802–7.

35. Eller JJ, Wolff S. Skin peeling and scarification. JAMA 1941; 116: 934–8.

36. Alster TS, West TB. Resurfacing of atrophic facial acne scars with a high-energy, pulsed carbon dioxide laser. Dermatol Surg 1996; 22: 151–5.

37. Walia S, Alster TS. Prolonged clinical and histological effects from laser resurfacing of atrophic acne scars. Dermatol Surg 1999; 25: 926–30.

38. Jeong TJ, Kye YC. Resurfacing of pitted facial acne scars with a long-pulsed Er:YAG laser. Dermatol Surg 2001; 27: 107–10.

39. Cho SI, Kim YC. Treatment of atrophic facial scars with combined use of high-energy pulsed CO2 laser and Er:YAG laser. Dermatol Surg 1999; 25: 959–64.

40. Orentreich DS, Orentreich N. Subcutaneous incisionless (subcision) surgery for the correction of depressed scars and wrinkles. Dermatol Surg 1995; 21: 543–9.

41. Arouete J. Correction of depressed scars on the face by a method of elevation. J Dermatol Surg Oncol 1976; 2: 337–9.

42. Field LM. Razorblade sculpturing and razabrasion versus scalpel sculpturing and scalpel abrasion. Dermatol Surg 1995; 21: 185–6.

43. Klein AW. Implantation techniques for injectable collagen. J Am Acad Dermatol 1983; 9: 224–8.

44. Selmanowitz VJ, Orentreich N. Medical grade fluid silicone: a monographic review. J Dermatol Surg Oncol 1977; 3: 597–611.

45. Fulton JE, Silverton K. Resurfacing the acne-scarred face. Dermatol Surg 1999; 25: 353–9.

46. Moritz DL. Surgical corrections of acne scars. Dermatol Nurs 1992; 4: 291–9.

47. Fernandes D. Minimally invasive percutaneous collagen induction, oral and maxillofacial. Surg Clin N Am 2005; 17: 51–63.

48. Jacob CI, Dover JS, Kaminer MS. Acne scarring: a classification system and review of treatment options. J Am Acad Dermatol 2001; 45(1): 109–17.

49. Whang KK, Lee M. The principle of a three-staged operation in the surgery of acne-scars. J Am Acad Dermatol 1999; 40: 95–7.

50. Stagnone JJ. Chemabrasion, a combined technique of chemical peeling and dermabrasion. J Dermatol Surg Oncol 1977; 3: 217–9.

51. Stal S, Hamilton S, Spira M. Surgical treatment of acne scars. Clin Plast Surg 1987; 14: 261–76.

52. Orentreich D, Orentreich N. Acne scar revision update. Dermatol Clin 1987; 5: 359–68.

53. Alster TS, West TB. Treatment of scars: a review. Ann Plast Surg 1997; 39: 418–32.

54. Solish N, Raman M, Pollack SV. Approaches to acne scarring: a review. J Cutan Med Surg 1998; 2: 24–32.

55. Kadunc BV, Trindade de Almeida AR. Surgical treatment of facial acne scars based on morphologic classification: a Brazilian experience. Dermatol Surg 2003; 29(12): 1200–9.

56. Strauss JS. Sebaceous glands. In: Fitzpatrick TB, Eisen AZ, Wolff K, Freedburg IM, Austen KF, editors. Dermatology in general medicine. 4th edition. New York: McGraw-Hill; 1993: 709–26.

57. Goodman GJ. Postacne scarring: a review of its pathophysiology and treatment. Dermatol Surg 2000; 26: 857–71.

58. Webster GF, Leyden JJ, Nilsson UR. Complement activation in acne vulgaris: consumption of complement by comedones. Infect Immun 1979; 26: 183–6.

59. Tucker SB, Rogers RS, Winkelmann RK et al. Inflammation in acne vulgaris: leukocyte attraction and cytotoxicity by comedonal material. J Invest Dermatol 1980; 74: 21–5.

60. Knutson D. Ultrastructural observations in acne vulgaris: the normal sebaceous follicle and acne lesions. J Invest Dermatol 1974; 62: 288–307.

61. Erlich HP, Desmouliere A, Cohen IK et al. Morphological and immunohistochemical differences between keloid and hypertrophic scar. Am J Pathol 1994; 145 (1): 105–13.

62. Goodman GJ, Baron JA. The management of postacne scarring. Dermatol Surg 2007; 33: 1175–88.

63. Patel N, Clement M. Selective nonablative treatment of acne scarring with 585 nm flashlamp pulsed dye laser. Dermatol Surg 2002; 28: 942–5.

64. Alster TS. Improvement of erythematous and hypertrophic scars by the 585 nm flashlamp-pumped pulse dye laser. Ann Plast Surg 1994; 32: 186.

65. Lupton JR, Alster TS. Laser scar revision. Dermatol Clin 2002; 20: 55–65.

66. Bowes LE, Alster TS. Treatment of facial scarring and ulceration resulting from acne excorie with 585 nm pulsed dye laser irradiation and cognitive psychotherapy. Dermatol Surg 2004; 30: 934–8.

67. Stratigos AJ, Katsambas AD. Optimal management of recalcitrant disorders of hyperpigmentation in dark-skinned patients. Am J Clin Dermatol 2004; 5: 161–8.

68. Goldman MP. The use of hydroquinone with facial laser resurfacing. J Cutan Laser Ther 2000; 2: 73–7.

69. Cuce LC, Bertino MC, Scattone L, Birkenhauer MC. Tretinoin peeling. Dermatol Surg 2001; 27: 12–4.

70. Wang CM, Huang CL, Hu CT, Chan HL. The effect of glycolic acid on the treatment of acne in Asian skin. Dermatol Surg 1997; 23(1): 23–9.

71. Bekhor PS. The role of pulsed laser in the management of cosmetically significant pigmented lesions. Australas J Dermatol 1995; 36: 221–3.

72. Chan H. The use of lasers and intense pulsed light sources for the treatment of acquired pigmentary lesions in Asians. J Cosmet Laser Ther 2003; 5: 198–200.

73. Roxo RF, Sarmento DF, Kawalek AZ, Spencer JM. Successful treatment of a hypochromic scar with manual dermabrasion: case report. Dermatol Surg 2003; 29: 189–91.

74. Camirand A, Doucet J. Needle dermabrasion. Aesthetic Plast Surg 1997; 21: 48–51.

75. Boersma BR, Westerhof W, Bos JD. Repigmentation in vitiligo vulgaris by autologous minigrafting: results in nineteen patients. J Am Acad Dermatol 1995; 33: 990–5.

76. Falabella R, Arrunategui A, Barona MI, Alzate A. The minigrafting test for vitiligo: detection of stable lesions for melanocyte transplantation. J Am Acad Dermatol 1995; 33: 1061–2.

77. Mulekar SV. Long-term follow-up study of segmental and focal vitiligo treated by autologous, noncultured melanocyte-keratinocyte cell transplantation. Arch Dermatol 2004; 140: 1211–5.

78. Stoner ML, Wood FM. The treatment of hypopigmented lesions with cultured epithelial autograft. J Burn Care Rehabil 2000; 21: 50–4.

79. Treatment of depressed cutaneous scars with gelatin matrix implant. J Am Acad Dermatol 1987; 16: 1155–62.

80. Swinehart JM. Pocket grafting with dermal grafts: autologous collagen implants for permanent correction of cutaneous depressions. Am J Cosmet Surg 1995; 12: 321–31.

81. Goodman GJ. Blood Transfer: the use of autologous blood as a chromophore and tissue augmentation agent. Dermatol Surg 2001; 27: 857–62.

82. Stegman SJ, Tromovitch TA. Cosmetic dermatologic surgery.Chicago: Year Book Medical Publishers, 1984: 47–76.

83. Robertson KM. Acne vulgaris. Facial Plast Surg Clin North Am 2004; 12: 347–55.

84. Horst Liebl. Stimulation of cell growth: abstract reflection about Collagen Induction Therapy (CIT), A hypothesis for the mechanism of action of Collagen Induction Therapy using Micro-Needles, 1st edition February 2006, 2nd revision January 2007.

85. Manstein D, Herron GS, Sink RK et al. Fractional photothermolysis: a new concept for cutaneous remodeling using microscopic patterns of thermal injury. Lasers Surg Med 2004; 34: 426–38.

86. Kim KH, Geronemus RG. Nonablative laser and light therapies for skin rejuvenation. Arch Facial Plast Surg 2004; 6: 398–409.

87. Sadick NS, Schecter AK. A preliminary study of utilization of the 1320 nm Nd:YAG laser for the treatment of acne scarring. Dermatol Surg 2004; 30: 995–1000.

88. Chua SH, Ang P, Khoo LS, Goh CL. Nonablative 1450 nm diode laser in the treatment of facial atrophic acne scars in type IV to V Asian skin: a prospective clinical study. Dermatol Surg 2004; 30: 1287–91.

89. Tanzi EL, Alster TS. Comparison of a 1450 nm diode laser and a 1320 nm Nd: a prospective clinical and histologic study. Dermatol Surg 2004; 30: 152–7.

90. Chan HH, Lam LK, Wong DS et al. Use of 1,320 nm Nd:YAG laser for wrinkle reduction and the treatment of atrophic acne scarring in Asians. Lasers Surg Med 2004; 34: 98–103.

91. Goldberg DJ. Nonablative dermal remodeling (does it really work?). Arch Dermatol 2002; 138: 1366–7.

92. Goldberg D. Nonablative subsurface remodeling: clinical and histologic evaluation of a 1320 nm Nd:YAG laser. J Cutan Laser Ther 1999; 1: 153–7.

93. Trelles MA, Allones I, Luna R. Facial rejuvenation with a nonablative 1320 nm Nd:YAG laser: a preliminary clinical and histologic evaluation. Dermatol Surg 2001; 27: 111–6.

94. Menaker G, Wrone D, Williams R et al. Treatment of facial rhytides with a nonablative laser: a clinical and histologic study. Dermatol Surg 1999; 25: 440–4.

95. Fatemi A, Weiss MA, Weiss RA. Short-term histologic effects of nonablative resurfacing: results with a dynamically cooled millisecond-domain 1320 nm Nd:YAG laser. Dermatol Surg 2002; 28: 172–6.

96. Zisser M, Kaplan B, Moy RL. Surgical pearl: manual dermabrasion. J Am Acad Dermatol 1995; 33: 105–6.

97. Harris DR, Noodleman FR. Combining manual dermasanding with low strength trichloroacetic acid to improve actinically injured skin. J Dermatol Surg Oncol 1994; 20: 436–42.

98. Bridenstine JB, Dolezal JF. Standardizing chemical peel solution formulations to avoid mishaps: great fluctuations in actual concentrations of trichloroacetic acid. J Dermatol Surg Oncol 1994; 20: 813–6.

99. Zachary CB. Modulating the Er:YAG laser. Lasers Surg Med 2000; 26: 223–6.

100. McDaniel DH, Lord J, Ash K, Newman J. Combined CO2/erbium: YAG laser resurfacing of perioral rhytids and side to side comparison with carbon dioxide laser alone. Dermatol Surg 1999; 25: 285–93.

101. Collawn SS. Combination therapy: utilisation of CO2 and erbium: YAG lasers for skin resurfacing. Ann Plast Surg 1999; 42: 21–6.

102. Tope WD. Multi-electrode radiofrequency resurfacing of ex vivo human skin. Dermatol Surg 1999; 25: 348–52.

103. Burns RL, Carruthers A, Langtry JA, et al. Electrosurgical skin resurfacing: a new bipolar instrument. Dermatol Surg 1999; 25: 583–6.

104. West TB, Alster TS. Commentary (on electrosurgical resurfacing). Dermatol Surg 1999; 25: 586.

105. Alexiades-Armenakas MR. Laser skin tightening: Non-surgical alternative to the face-lift. J Drugs Dermatol 2006; 5: 295–6.

106. Jacobson LG, Alexiades-Armenakas MR, Bernstein L, Geronemus RG. Treatment of nasolabial folds and jowls with a non-invasive radiofrequency device. Arch Dermatol 2003; 139: 1313–20.

107. Hsu TS, Kaminer MS. The use of nonablative radiofrequency technology to tighten the lower face and neck. Semin Cutan Med Surg 2003; 22: 115–23.

108. Sadick N, Alexiades-Armenakas M, Bitter P, Hruza G, Mulholland S. Enhanced full-face skin rejuvenation using synchronous intense pulsed optical and conducted, bipolar radiofrequency energy (ELOS): Introducing selective radiophotothermolysis. J Drugs Dermatol 2005; 4: 181–6.

109. Doshi SN, Alster TS. Combination radiofrequency and diode laser for treatment of facial rhytides and skin laxity. J Cosmet Laser Ther 2005; 7: 11–5.

110. Alexiades-Armenakas MR. Unipolar versus bipolar radiofrequency for skin tightening and wrinkle reduction. Laser Surg Med 2007; 19: 21.

111. Alexiades-Armenakas MR. Laser-mediated photodynamic therapy. Clin Dermatol 2006; 24: 16–25.

112. Orentreich DS. Punch graft. In: Lask GP, Moy RL, eds. Principles and Techniques of Cutaneous Surgery. New York: McGraw-Hill, 1996: 283–95.

113. Johnson WC. Treatment of pitted scars: punch transplant technique. J Dermatol Surg Oncol 1986; 12: 260–5.

114. Lee JB, Chung WG, Kwahck H, Lee KH. Focal treatment of acne scars with trichloroacetic acid: chemical reconstruction of skin scars method. Dermatol Surg 2002; 28: 1017–21.

115. Ellenbogen R. Invited comment on autologous fat injection. Ann Plast Surg 1990; 24: 297.

116. Ersek RA. Transplantation of purified autologous fat: a 3-year follow up is disappointing. Plast Reconstr Surg 1991; 87: 219–27.

117. Coleman SR. Long-term survival of fat transplants: controlled demonstrations. Aesthetic Plast Surg 1995; 19: 421–5.

118. Eppley BL, Snyders RV Jr, Winkelmann T, Delfino JJ. Autologous facial fat transplantation: improved graft maintenance by microbead bioactivation. J Oral Maxillofac Surg 1992; 50: 477–82.

119. Pinski KS, Roenigk HH Jr. Autologous fat transplantation: long term follow-up. J Dermatol Surg Oncol 1992; 18: 179–82.

120. Signorini M, Clementoni MT. Clinical evaluation of a new self-drying silicone gel in the treatment of scars: a preliminary report. Aesthetic Plast Surg 2007; 31(2): 183–7.

121. Tandara AA, Mustoe TA. The role of the epidermis in the control of scarring: evidence for mechanism of action for silicone gel. J Plast Reconstr Aesthet Surg 2008; 22. [Epub ahead of print]

122. Lacarrubba F, Patania L, Perrotta R et al. An open-label pilot study to evaluate the efficacy and tolerability of a silicone gel in the treatment of hypertrophic scars using clinical and ultrasound assessments. J Dermatolog Treat 2008; 19(1): 50–3.

123. Reish RG, Eriksson E. Scar treatments: preclinical and clinical studies. J Am Coll Surg 2008; 2006(4): 719–30.

124. Durani P, Bayat A. Levels of evidence for the treatment of keloid disease. J Plast Reconstr Aesthet Surg 2008; 61(1): 4–17.

125. Atiyeh BS. Nonsurgical management of hypertrophic scars: evidence-based therapies, standard practices, and emerging methods. Aesthetic Plast Surg 2007; 31(5): 468–92.

126. Roques C, Téot L. The use of corticosteroids to treat keloids: a review. Int J Low Extrem Wounds 2008; 8. [Epub ahead of print]

127. Lebwohl M. From the literature. intralesional 5-FU in the treatment of hypertrophic scars and keloids: clinical experience. J Am Acad Dermatol 2000; 42: 677.

128. Uppal RS, Khan U, Kakar S et al. The effects of a single dose of 5-fluorouracil on keloid scars: a clinical trial of timed wound irrigation after extralesional excision. Plast Reconstr Surg 2001; 108: 1218–24.

129. Wendling J, Marchand A, Mauviel A, Verrecchia F. 5-Fluorouracil blocks transforming growth factor-beta-induced alpha 2 type I collagen gene (COL1A2) expression in human fibroblasts viac-Jun NH2-terminal kinase/activator protein-1 activation. Mol Pharmacol 2003; 64: 707–13.

130. Alster TS, Williams CM. Treatment of keloid sternotomy scars with 585 nm flashlamp-pumped pulsed-dye laser. Lancet 1995; 345: 1198–2000.

131. Manuskiatti W, Fitzpatrick RE. Treatment response of keloidal and hypertrophic sternotomy scars: comparison among intralesional corticosteroid, 5-fluorouracil, and 585 nm flashlamp-pumped pulsed-dye laser treatments. Arch Dermatol 2002; 138: 1149–55.

132. Jalali M, Bayat A. Current use of steroids in management of abnormal raised skin scars. Surgeon 2007; 5: 175–80.

133. Rusciani L, Paradisi A, Alfano C et al. Cryotherapy in the treatment of keloids. J Drugs Dermatol 2006; 5(7): 591–5.

134. Annacontini L, Parisi D, Maiorella A et al. Long-term follow-up in the treatment of keloids by combined surgical excision and immediate postoperative adjuvant irradiation. Plast Reconstr Surg 2008; 121(2): 700–1.

135. Arons JA. The results of surgical excision and adjuvant irradiation for therapy-resistant keloids: a prospective clinical outcome study. Plast Reconstr Surg 2008; 121(2): 685–6.

136. Copcu E, Sivrioglu N, Oztan Y. Combination of surgery and intralesional verapamil injection in the treatment of the keloid. J Burn Care Rehabil 2004; 25: 1–7.

137. Berman B, Villa A. Imiquimod 5% cream for keloid management. Dermatol Surg 2003; 29: 1050–1.

138. Holland DB, Jeremy AH, Roberts SG et al. Inflammation in acne scarring: a comparison of the responses in lesions from patients prone and not prone to scar. Br J Dermatol 2004; 150: 72–81.

139. Rosen L. Antiangiogenic strategies and agents in clinical trials. Oncologist 2000; 5: 20–7.

140. Cockerill GW, Gamble JR, Vadas MA. Angiogenesis: models and modulators. Int Rev Cytol 1995; 159: 113–60.

141. Gillard JA, Reed MW, Buttle D et al. Matrix metalloproteinase activity and immunohistochemical profile of matrix metalloproteinase-2 and -9 and tissue inhibitor of metalloproteinase-1 during human dermal wound healing. Wound Repair Regen 2004; 12: 295–304.

142. Dang CM, Beanes SR, Lee H et al. Scarless fetal wounds are associated with an increased matrix metalloproteinase-to-tissuederived inhibitor of metalloproteinase ratio. Plast Reconstr Surg 2003; 111: 2273–85.

143. Tortora G, Melisi D, Ciardiello F. Angiogenesis: a target for cancer therapy. Curr Pharm Des 2004; 10: 11–26.

Index